THE FAT-TO-MUSCLE DIET

THE FAT-TO-MUSCLE DIET

Victoria Zak
Cris Carlin, M.S., R.D.
Peter Vash, M.D., M.P.H.

G. P. Putnam's Sons
New York

TO
Leona Zak;
Teri and Dan Carlin;
&
George, Virginia, Barbara,
and Stephen Vash

Acknowledgments: The authors would like to thank John Brockman and Katinka Matson, our agents, and E. Stacy Creamer, our editor. And special thanks to George L. Blackburn, M.D., Ph.D., in recognition of his pioneer research in the field and his influence on our work.

G. P. Putnam's Sons
Publishers Since 1838
200 Madison Avenue
New York, NY 10016

Library of Congress Cataloging-in-Publication Data

Zak, Victoria.
    The fat to muscle diet.

    1. Reducing diets. 2. Metabolism. 3. Reducing
exercises. I. Carlin, Cris. II. Vash, Peter.
III. Title.
RM222.2.Z35   1987   613.2'5   86-25517
ISBN 0-399-13231-7

Printed in the United States of America
20 19 18 17 16 15 14 13 12

Contents

1. Introduction   7

2. Measuring Your Fat-to-Muscle Ratio   11
   Body Fat Standards   13

3. You Are What You Burn   14
   Resting Metabolic Rate   14
   Physical Activity   17
   Thermic Effect of Food   18
   Fat Addicts   20
   Better Thermic Burn   21
   Preserving Your Burn   22
   Your Body Bank   23

4. Fat-to-Muscle Diet: The Most Power for the Fewest Calories   24
   Your Daily Diet Tray   26
   Your Daily Diet Hotplates   26
   A Perfect Thermic Day   27
   Your Fat-to-Muscle Food Lists   28

5. The Burn 1 and Burn 2 Diets   30
   Burn 1   30
   Creating Meal Menus   34
   Menus and Recipes   37
   Burn 2   38

6. Starting Your Diet   44
   Choosing Your Goal   44
   Matching Your Diet to Your Goal   45

7. Your Fat-to-Muscle Calendar   48
   Setting Yourself Up Right   52
   Figuring Degree of Fat Trouble   52

8. **Thermic Action: Your Exercise Hotlist**   55
   Action Aerobics   56
   Marvelous Machines   59
   Skill Sport Aerobics   66
   Why You Need Exercise from Day 1 of
      Your Diet   68
   Cardiovascular Conditioning   70
   Taking Your Target Heart Rate   71
   Warm-Ups   73
   Cool-Downs   75
   Selecting the Right Shoes   76
   How Fat Are Your Favorite Athletes?   77

9. **Behavior Modification**   81
   Ideal Body *What?*   82
   Beating the Body Weight Trap   82
   Loosening Up in Your Clothes   83
   Tracking Your Progress   83
   Your Scale   84
   Water: Keeping Your Fat Removal Moving   85
   Gaining Mental Muscle   87
   Creating Your Diet Environment   89
   Eating Low-Fat   92
   Why You Eat What You Eat   93
   Emergency Thermic Boosters   102
   Relief: Exercises for Relaxation, Tension
      Release, and Stress Reduction   105
   Facing Up to Stress   108
   Rewards   109
   How to Handle a Diet Breakdown   111

10. **Maintenance: Keeping Your Low-Fat Status**   115
    for Life
    How to Eat for Maintenance   116
    Counting Your Daily Fat Grams   117
    Fail-Safe Maintenance   118

11. **Burn 1 Menus**   120

12. **Burn 2 Menus**   131

13. **Thermic Burn Recipes: Gourmet Dining on a**   142
    Thermic Diet

    Appendix: Fat-Gram Counter   163

ONE

INTRODUCTION

This program is about *heat*—the heat you need to burn more calories than you store. It's calorie *burning*, not calorie cutting, that gives you the metabolic power you've been missing on other programs.

When you go on a diet, what do you want? To be thinner, firmer, fitter, and to feel better about yourself. Do you want it to last? Then you need a diet that does more than cut your calories or juggle your foods around in strange combinations that jeopardize your health. You need to drive up the power of your metabolism, improving your ability to burn calories.

Your metabolism is not an inner-body thermostat designed to keep you fat. It's an intricate and marvelous process that keeps you burning calories even when you sleep— even when you eat. Its power is measured in terms of heat, and you can increase that power.

By boosting your metabolism to produce more heat, you can burn calories stronger and longer, remove stored fat, lose your excess weight, and avoid gaining it back. You reach your desired weight in excellent physical shape with your fat-to-muscle ratio in better body balance *inside*. This is the ratio that counts—it keeps your fat problems from returning. You also feel the benefits of a balanced fat-to-muscle body with more energy, stamina, and tone, and a lean appearance that broadcasts your health.

The Fat-to-Muscle Diet is a revolution in weight loss. You lose *only fat*, and you increase your lean muscle tissue— the metabolic "hothouses" where your calorie-burning process is activated. With better fat-to-muscle balance at the end of your diet, you become a stronger calorie-burning machine, which means you can eat more calories without gaining your weight back. Regardless of your age, sex, or weight, you can boost your calorie-burning power by dieting to fix your fat-to-muscle ratio.

The reason 95 percent of today's diets fail to keep your weight off is that they cause you to lose muscle tissue along with your fat. These muscle losses are critical. They slow down your metabolism and reduce your calorie-burning power. They leave you drawn, listless, and less healthy, and—most surprising of all—they can leave you "fatter" on the inside than before you started dieting. You can "look thinner" on the outside, and fit smaller sizes, but you won't stay thin for long because of muscle loss. Fat will come back faster than it left. This is called the yo-yo syndrome— a cycle of losing-gaining, losing-gaining that you will not be able to stop, because of muscle loss. Here's a typical dieter's story:

Dieting Wrong Is Worse than Not Dieting at All

115 lbs: 25 percent fat–75 percent muscle. A 5-foot-3-inch healthy 25-year-old woman weighs 115 pounds. Her proportion of fat to muscle (lean body mass*) is normal. She has 29 pounds of fat (25 percent) and 86 pounds of lean body mass. From this point on, she eats 100 more calories per day than she burns in daily activity. At the end of 2 years, our 27-year-old woman has gained approximately 20 pounds.

135 lbs: 34 percent fat–66 percent muscle. She now weighs 135 pounds, but her body composition has changed. She has approximately 46 pounds of fat (34 percent) and 89 pounds of lean body mass. Summer is approaching and she wants to look good in her bathing suit. She wants to lose those 20 pounds. She can follow a sound diet of 1,000– 1,200 calories per day, expecting weight loss of about 2 pounds per week. Wanting to lose weight faster, she follows one of the popular rapid weight loss plans that promises

---

Lean body mass is the scientific term for muscle. Your lean body mass includes muscle, water, and bones, but most of it is muscle.

she can lose 20 pounds in 6–8 weeks, which she does by crash dieting on less than 800 calories per day. No mystery or miracle about it—she eats less than she burns and she loses weight. But there's a price she doesn't know she's paying.

115 lbs: 31 percent fat–69 percent muscle. The 20 pounds she loses are not all fat. She loses only 10 pounds of fat, 5 pounds of water, and 5 pounds of muscle. Her body composition is altered by the diet. Back at her original 115 pounds, she is now *fatter*, with 36 pounds of fat (31 percent and 79 pounds of lean body mass. She now has less muscle than she had when she was 25, and more fat. When summer is over, she becomes less active and falls back into her old eating habits. Slowly but surely, she regains the 20 pounds she lost. But here's where the real trouble starts.

135 lbs: 38 percent fat–62 percent muscle. Something drastic happens to her when she gains her 20 pounds back. The 20 pounds she regains are mostly fat. She regains 5 pounds of water and 15 pounds of fat. She has 51 pounds of fat and 84 pounds of lean body mass. If she loses weight again by cutting her calories back, and the cycle is repeated three more times, she can come down to her original 115 pounds, but her body composition will be dangerously changed from muscle loss.

115 lbs: 40 percent fat–60 percent muscle. Our female dieter, now 30 years old, is the victim of her unorthodox weight-loss practices. She has a metabolically reduced body system, which needs fewer calories to maintain herself. She has 46 pounds of fat (40 percent) and 69 pounds of lean body mass. On the outside, she looks slim, but on the inside, she qualifies as high-fat obese. If her metabolic needs are reduced by only 100 calories per day, because of her high-fat body composition, without increasing her calories, she will still gain 10 pounds per year.

At this point, she says:

"What's wrong with me? Why do I gain weight so easily, barely touching food, when my girlfriend of the same height, weight, and age can eat what she wants and not gain a pound? I must have a slow metabolism."

She is correct.

Her reduced amount of lean muscle tissue and slowed metabolic rate will keep her gaining fat, even when she diligently controls her calories.*

More than any other factor, drastic dieting is a serious threat to your metabolism, because of muscle loss. This also seriously reduces your enjoyment of life, limiting the amount of calories you can eat without gaining weight.

What kind of diet causes you to lose muscle?

• Rapid-weight-loss plans.
• Unsupervised calorie restriction under 800 calories per day.
• One- or two-food combination diets.
• Formula diets without medical supervision.
• Pills and appetite suppressants for starving.
• Diets without nutritional balance.
• Diets without exercise.

Since muscle is lost proportionately from every part of your body, including the vital organ of your heart, muscle is something you cannot afford to lose on a diet. Muscle is what you should *gain.*

The Fat-to-Muscle Diet will turn your fat problem into a muscle advantage by the end of your program. When you lose only fat and gain valuable muscle tissue, you can reverse the mistakes you've made in the past with bad dieting and poor nutrition. A diet is an investment in your future self. When you make the right investment, you get the right payoff.

A metabolic expert once referred to metabolism as the "fine-tuned mechanism of your internal calorie regulator." When it's tuned, it works to keep you lean.

---

*The material in this section is adapted from "The Yo-Yo Syndrome," G. L. Blackburn, M.D., Ph.D., K. N. Pavlou, Sc.D., and V. Zak, in *RxWeight Control*, vol. 2, no. 5, June–July 1984.

TWO

MEASURING YOUR FAT-TO-MUSCLE RATIO

How much fat and how much muscle do you have?

The simple system below will allow you to make a reasonable at-home estimate of your percent of body fat. Once you have your percent of body fat, subtract that from 100 and you have your muscle rating.

Charting Your Starting Point

Women

1. Use an ordinary tape measure and measure your hip line in inches (around the widest part of your pantyline and buttocks).
2. Mark a dot on the grid entitled HIP GIRTH at the point of your hip measurement.
3. Take your height in inches and mark a dot on the HEIGHT grid at the point of your height measurement.
4. Draw a line connecting the dots from HIP GIRTH to HEIGHT.

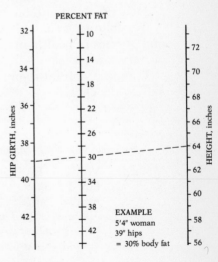

PERCENT FAT

HIP GIRTH, inches

HEIGHT, inches

EXAMPLE
5'4" woman
39" hips
= 30% body fat

Men

1. Use an ordinary tape measure and measure your waist circumference (around the biggest bulge on your waist).
2. Mark a dot on the grid entitled **WAIST GIRTH** at the point of your waist measurement.
3. Take your weight in pounds and mark a dot on the **BODY WEIGHT** grid at the point of your total weight.
4. Draw a line connecting the dots from **WAIST GIRTH** to **BODY WEIGHT**.

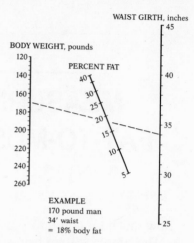

EXAMPLE
170 pound man
34' waist
= 18% body fat

Where the connecting line crosses the **PERCENT FAT** grid is your approximate percent of body fat. Subtract that from 100 and you have your muscle rating.

Our thanks to Jack Wilmore, Ph.D., for giving us permission to reprint his valuable chart.

How much fat and how much muscle should you have?

The following chart shows fat-to-muscle ratios for varying degrees of health and fitness from very-high-fat obese to very-low-fat lean.

Compare your fat-to-muscle status to find out where you fall on the chart.

	Body Status	Percent Body Fat	Percent Lean Body Mass
Women	Very-Low-Fat *Lean*	10–17%	90–83%
	Low-Fat *Slim*	17–22	83–78
	Average-Fat *Ideal*	22–25	78–75
	Above-Average *Trouble*	25–29	75–71
	High-Fat *Overfat*	29–35	71–65
	Very-High-Fat *Obese*	35 +	65 −

	Body Status	Percent Body Fat	Percent Lean Body Mass
Men	Very-Low Fat *Lean*	7–10%	93–90%
	Low-Fat *Slim*	10–15	90–85
	Average-Fat *Ideal*	15–18	85–82
	Above-Average *Trouble*	18–20	82–80
	High-Fat *Overfat*	20–25	80–75
	Very-High-Fat *Obese*	25+	75–

Body Fat Standards

The ideal percent of body fat is 16–19 percent for men and 22–25 percent for women. People with up to 5 percent more body fat than this are "overweight." Those with greater deviations—25 percent for men and 35 percent for women—are obese. Since women have a greater percentage of essential fat—approximately 13 percent for women compared to 3 percent for men—women are usually 7–10 percent fatter than men.

Significant body composition differences between men and women don't have to be the rule. If a male and female of the same age and height continue with the same physical training after their teens and both eat nutritious, calorie-balanced diets, body composition differences are less pronounced. Women athletes, for instance, average 12–20 percent body fat, instead of the average 25 percent.

However, women should not try to lower their percentage of body fat to the equivalent *Lean* percent for men. Striving for the fatless figure can be carried to an unhealthy extreme, resulting in physiological changes in the female body. Some female athletes whose percent of body fat drops too low experience loss of menstruation and face an increased risk of osteoporosis.

The ideal is to strive for a lower percent of body fat than you now have, preferably in the *Ideal* or *Slim* range, in order to maximize your body's calorie-burning power.

THREE

YOU ARE WHAT YOU BURN

Body fat is stored calories. To lose your stored fat, you have to burn more calories than you eat by driving up the heat production in the three main burners of your metabolism:

	Percent of Calorie Burn
Resting Metabolic Rate	60%
Physical Activity	25
Thermic Effect of Food	15

Your resting metabolic rate, physical activity, and the thermic effect of your food are all heat-producing, or *thermic* processes. Together, they build your calorie-burning power.

RESTING METABOLIC RATE

Most of the calories you use are burned by your *metabolic rate*, often called *resting metabolism*, since it is measured in a resting state. On the average, your metabolic rate requires 60–70 percent of your total calories just to run its shop. This is the energy required to keep your heart pumping, brain active, organs functioning, lungs breathing, down to the simplest act, like keeping your eyelids blinking so you can wink and flirt. It's the level of energy needed to sustain your body's vital functions.

To figure the power of your metabolic rate, use the following formula: Your weight in pounds ÷ 2.2 (kilograms) × 24 (hours in a day). This will show you how many calories are currently burned by your metabolic rate each day.

Your metabolic rate is the biggest burner in your metabolism. You cannot afford to compromise it during a diet. And yet that's exactly what happens if you cut your calories without simultaneously increasing your burning power. When you only cut calories, you run right into a metabolic trap.

Most dieters think of calories as little fat machines in food. But calories are *heat* you eat. When you reduce the heat you eat (calories), your metabolic rate reduces the heat it generates to burn those calories. You are eating less, but burning less too.

Studies on normal and obese people who followed very-low-calorie diets for several weeks showed a 15–30-percent *drop* in their metabolic rates.

This means that you burn *fewer* calories during the course of your diet, when you only cut calories. It also means that you can eat fewer calories without gaining weight at the end of your diet, because of your lowered metabolic rate. This is one of the main reasons that calorie-cutting diets fail over and over again.

A decrease in your metabolic rate can lead to a real problem midway in your diet, or in the final stretch, when you are hovering around your ideal weight. You reach a plateau, where you stop losing weight as fast, or you stop losing weight entirely. If you have ever reached a plateau on a diet, you know how frustrating this can be.

A plateau occurs when you stop losing weight *before you reach your ideal goal* and you can't get below that weight. It's the danger zone for diet breaks. Most diet books don't even talk about plateaus, letting you go off on your own to face them alone. Or if you're told anything at all, you are asked to be patient. Or you're told that this is a common phenomenon (but you aren't told why), and if you stick with your calorie-cutting, you'll start losing weight again later. Not true, if you are losing too much muscle and lowering your burning power.

Plateaus don't have to be deadlocks. You can do something about them, but the worst thing to do is cut your calories back further, risking another decrease in your metabolic rate and your ability to burn calories.

When your metabolic rate drops by 10–15 percent because of calorie restriction during a diet, you have to take action to regain that 15 percent. It's only logical. You have to give yourself something back—at least 15 percent more *heat* production to offset your loss.

The *giveback* will come from aerobic exercise, another thermic process.

Exercise is heat producing, and metabolic rate has been proven to increase by 10–15 percent during aerobic activity. By adding an aerobic charge to your diet at the right time and in the right amount, you offset the loss of heat by your metabolism caused by calorie-cutting. In addition, you get a bonus! Your metabolic rate stays higher up to 48 hours after you stop exercising. Studies on morning-after metabolic rate measured a 4.7 percent increase, even after sleeping.

When you compare dieting with exercise to dieting without, it will drive our thermic point home. Dieters who ate low-calorie diets *without* exercise showed a 20 percent drop in their metabolic rates. With this metabolic decrease, they also showed dramatic differences in the *quality* of weight they lost. Non-exercising dieters not only burn calories slower, but also lose some of the vital lean muscle tissue that we've been talking about.

In a recent study, dieters were given the same 1,000 calorie diets and separated into exercise and nonexercise groups. At the end of their programs, the nonexercisers had lost a total of 18 pounds—*but 7 pounds of muscle were lost,* and only 11 pounds of fat. On the other hand, the exercisers lost a total of 19 pounds—and 23 pounds of fat were lost, while 4 pounds of muscle were gained. As a result, the exercisers had better fat-to-muscle ratios and better burning power at the end of their program, while the nonexercisers were left with inferior fat-to-muscle bodies and lower burning power.

Exerciser	Nonexerciser
1,000 calories per day	1,000 calories per day
19 lbs total weight loss	18 lbs total weight loss
23 lbs *fat* lost	11 lbs *fat* lost
4 lbs *lean muscle* gained	7 lbs *lean muscle* lost

The material in this section is adapted from "The Yo-Yo Syndrome," G. L. Blackburn, M.D., Ph.D., K. N. Pavlou, Sc.D., and V. Zak, in *RxWeight Control*, vol. 2, no. 5, June–July 1984.

Where do you want to be on your diet? Burning your calories too slowly, facing a plateau that you might not get over, heading for diet failure from frustration? Why settle for that, when you can slide over plateaus, steadily burn fat, and increase your lean muscle to burn better, heading toward a higher calorie maximum at maintenance.

That's why you must add exercise to your diet.

Dieting without exercise is simply too risky to try, since it can lead to muscle loss and cause an imbalance in your body composition.

The aerobic factor in your diet boosts your metabolism and burns fat steadily by increasing your calorie-burning power. It's the first step to fine-tuning your internal calorie regulator—your metabolism.

PHYSICAL ACTIVITY

In metabolic terms, *physical activity* does not mean the same thing as planned aerobic activity. It refers to the normal day-to-day movement of a moderately active person going about the business of living. You get up, get dressed, work, lift things, put them down, walk around, do housework, make business deals, go out in the evening, and so forth. All of this is part of physical activity. Routine activity burns 25 percent of your total calories, if you are moderately active. However, most people are not active enough to reach the maximum calorie-burning potential for physical activity.

To boost your metabolism to burn better and longer to get rid of your stored fat, you need an extra "kick" from physical activity. We could suggest that you increase your normal daily activity and climb more stairs, bend over more, or take up an active hobby such as gardening, but we can't be sure you'll do enough exercise to burn the calories you need. Routine activities are not easy to plan. You have to sit down and figure out how many calories you burn during your current daily activity and what you would need to do to *burn* an extra 200–300 calories per day. And while you are sitting down doing all that calculating, you're not up and around and active!

So we did it for you. We added the extra "kick" to your exercise program. All you have to do is follow your Fat-to-Muscle Diet Calendar, and it's already worked into your day. In the meantime, each time you take the stairs instead of an elevator, or park your car farther from your door and walk the extra distance, you are adding to the boost, getting a better metabolism with better calorie-burning power.

THERMIC EFFECT OF FOOD

This is the most exciting part of your Fat-to-Muscle Diet. You are going to learn to eat *thermically*, in order to increase your calorie burn from eating. Remember, calories are heat you eat. When you eat the "hotter" calories—the ones that are more thermic—you burn more calories by the simple art of eating. Your metabolic rate rises in response to food in order to digest, absorb, and use the nutrients in those foods. This produces more heat. *You burn while you eat.* This heat production is called the *thermic effect of food,* and it can burn up to 15 percent of your total calories.

All foods do not produce the same thermic effect. Some are *hot,* some are not. You can eat 2,000 calories per day and burn up to 300 of those calories simply because you are eating the hotter, more thermic foods. That's the equivalent of four slices of bread per day that you could burn off by eating properly. When it comes to cutting calories for a diet, thermic eating is a real boost, because you can eat *more* food and burn better as a result. This makes it less likely that you will feel deprived of food during a diet or eat as if you are starving, or dread the whole idea of a diet. Dieting can be fun again, and food can be a friend, not an enemy.

Carbohydrates and protein are thermic, *but fat is not.* In fact, the thermic effect of fat is so low that your metabolism flickers instead of flames. The thermic responses of test animals who were fed a high-fat diet were so low that researchers concluded it was as if the animals hadn't eaten at all.

Fat in food has a profile that is already very similar to that of the fat found in your body. This makes fat metabolically prone to storage. To turn 200 calories of food fat into body fat, you burn only 3 percent of the total calories, or 6 little calories. The remaining 97 percent of those 200 calories—194 calories of fat—are readily available to be padded onto your thighs or added to your spare tire. It's very easy to eat 200 extra calories of fat. That's 1½ tablespoons of butter or oil. You can absorb that amount of fat in 25 small french fries that you can eat in a snap! If you do that every day, and don't burn if off, you can gain a pound of fat every 20 days.

The average American eats 40 percent of his or her total calories as fat. On a 2,000-calorie diet with 800 calories of fat, that leaves 776 fat calories a day that are in the right state to be stored. And you only burn 24 of the 800 fat calories to prepare that fat for storage.

The same problems occur in dieting. If you are on a diet with a limited amount of calories—say, 1,200 calories—and you eat 40 percent of those calories as dietary fat, you have 466 fat calories per day that prefer to be stored.

Because of fat's low thermic effect, you can defeat your weight loss efforts by eating too much fat during a diet. You can exercise regularly, but if you eat a high-fat diet that is thermically poor, you might not lose weight, or you might lose weight too slowly to keep you interested in your diet for long.

We did some serious calculating to try to help you understand the results of eating a high-fat, thermically poor diet, as opposed to a lower-fat, more thermic diet. We compared the thermic effects of eating a 40-percent fat diet with those of a 20-percent fat diet, with both diets totaling 2,000 calories. Here's what we found: If you eat 40 percent fat in your diet, you burn about 84 fewer calories per day than if you eat 20 percent fat in your diet. This adds up to 588 fewer calories burned per week, and 30,576 fewer calories burned per year from your reduced thermic response. That's 9 pounds of fat per year that you don't burn, or 9 pounds per year you *gain!* All because of the low thermic effect of fat.

FAT ADDICTS

One of the secondary characteristics of fat makes it very difficult to control on a casual basis, without taking serious steps to combat it.

Fat can increase your preference for sweets and more fats. Studies of college students showed that the more fat they ate, the less they were able to distinguish between sweets and fats. In fact, they actually preferred fatter and fatter formulas, while their tolerance for sweets was limited. This led to the theory that behind your sweet tooth is the phantom fat tooth that leads you to more sweets and fats.

In laboratory studies, normal-weight animals were offered two diet choices: a supermarket diet high in fat and sugar OR low-fat lab chow. What did the animals go for? You guessed it. They chose the fat-dense diet over their lab chow and proceeded to gain 269 percent more weight than the ones that were kept on low-fat lab chow.

Since eating fat leads to eating more fat and having less control over sweets, fat has all the earmarks of an *addictive* substance. Fat's addictive nature makes it very hard to remove from your diet without a serious program to break fat's hold over your life.

The Fat-to-Muscle Diet has a built-in plan of attack against fat. In the first few weeks, you eliminate all fats from your diet, except the hidden ones, in order to break your affinity for fat. As you become less dependent on fat, you gradually reintroduce fat into your diet, when your body is in better shape to handle the burning of fat. Also, you get a special maintenance bonus! A fat-gram counter, complete with over 300 foods, portion sizes, calories, percentage of total calories as fat, and our very own precalculated food fat rating system.

You can choose low-fat foods at a glance! No more guesswork about fats hidden in foods. You can stay low-fat for life!

BETTER THERMIC BURN

Carbohydrates are thermic foods. You burn more calories eating carbohydrates than eating fat.

To turn carbohydrates into body fat is very complicated since they are long-chain molecules. They trigger a chain reaction for digestion that takes them through more metabolic steps before they are absorbed. To turn 200 calories of carbohydrates into body fat, you burn about 23 percent of your total calories, compared to fat's 3 percent. This means that 46 out of every 200 carbohydrate calories burn off, while fat burns off only 6 calories. If you compare a

1,200-calorie diet with 40 percent fat to one with 40 percent carbohydrates, you'll find carbohydrates thermically burning 110 calories for eating and processing, while fat only burns 14 calories.

Think of how thermic you can be by raising the level of carbohydrates in your diet to 50–55 percent, while simultaneously cutting fat to avoid its lower thermic effect. In addition, carbohydrates are not like fat, in a profile for easy storage. By the time carbohydrates get through your system, most of your remaining carbohydrates are burned off.

Carbohydrates get turned into glycogen as they are processed, and you can only store half a pound of glycogen in your muscles and liver. But you can store unlimited pounds of fat in cells that expand to accommodate more fat. To get the full picture, you can store enough fat in your body to compensate for two to three months of starvation, but *one* aerobic workout can deplete your carbohydrate stores.

This is not to suggest that you can't get fat from overeating carbohydrates. Anything eaten to excess will store as fat. It's just more difficult with carbohydrates, and you can use this power to your advantage to burn fat. However, don't think for a minute that eating carbohydrates *alone* is the secret to successful weight loss. If you don't balance your diet with protein, you can lose the very thing we're working so hard to save—your valuable body protein in the form of lean muscle tissue!

PRESERVING YOUR BURN

Protein is *essential* in your diet to preserve your muscle tissue. If your body does not get enough protein in your diet, it will go after the protein in your muscles to burn for energy. Therefore, a diet without sufficient protein will only defeat your fat-to-muscle balance in the end. But beware! More protein is not better.

Proteins have a thermic effect similar to that of carbohydrates, and they burn while you eat. In fact, protein packs the biggest thermic punch, but there's a catch! The majority of high-protein foods are also high in fat, which reduces your overall thermic power. Since there are hidden fats in proteins, you can increase your fat intake without knowing it by eating high-fat proteins. To get the best thermic burn, you have to be selective about your proteins. You need 25–30 percent of your calories as protein when you are dieting, but only the most thermic proteins, which are the ones that are lowest in fat.

If you eat too much protein on your diet, you can create a calcium imbalance, since high-protein diets have been linked to calcium leeching from your bones. Protein-rich foods such as red meats are usually high in cholesterol, and any excess protein will simply store as fat.

YOUR BODY BANK

Taking all of this information to the body bank, in order to increase the thermic effect of your food, you need a diet that is carbohydrate-rich, low-fat, and balanced in protein. To burn calories better, you can't afford to cut your calories indiscriminately, because you will sacrifice more than nutrients. When you are adjusting your food for fat loss, you are on a tight fuel budget. Food is the fuel you need for stamina, daily energy, and disease prevention. You can't bet on fruit alone, or carbohydrates alone, or protein alone, for one more reason than the very vital matters of your heart, mind, muscle, bones, and general well-being—you'll burn less fat.

FOUR

FAT-TO-MUSCLE DIET: THE MOST POWER FOR THE FEWEST CALORIES

The Fat-to-Muscle Diet is a system that has built-in nutrients from Vitamin A to Zinc. It's the most nutrient-dense diet you can get on a 1,000-calorie-per-day plan, packing the most possible nutrients into the fewest possible calories. It improves your health while you burn fat. It protects your muscle while you burn fat. It's the foundation of sound dieting that will teach you how to burn while you eat, and how to eat right for life. No more worry about dehydration, dizziness, or physical weakness following a diet. The power is packed in your food, with all of the nutrients kicked in together to burn stronger and longer:

- 50–55 percent of your calories will come from nutrient-rich carbohydrates to increase your thermic response.

- 25–30 percent of your calories will come from high-quality, low-fat protein to protect your muscles while you burn fat and increase your thermic response.
- 15–20 percent of your calories will come from fat. This is your fat maximum to minimize fat's low thermic response and insure that you get the best body fat burn.

You will also receive the following protective benefits:

- 800 mg per day of calcium to preserve your bone strength (plain yogurt is your best source of calcium).
- 30 grams per day of fiber to satisfy your hunger and keep your food moving through your system.
- A vitamin and mineral supplement as fail-safe nutrient insurance.

In addition to maximizing your thermic power, this diet:

- Meets 100 percent of your RDA's for good nutrition during dieting.
- Meets the American Cancer Society's recommendations and the American Heart Association's guidelines for low-fat dietary intake for disease prevention, including hypertension, diabetes, heart disease, bowel cancer for men, and breast cancer for women.
- Meets protein requirements from the Center for Nutritional Research for muscle protection during dieting.
- Reverses a dangerous dieting trend of the last decade, which shows Americans eating too much fat and too few complex carbohydrates.
- Keeps you calcium-supplied to ward off osteoporosis.

Goodbye Fat. Hello Muscle. The power is packed in your food.

YOUR DAILY DIET TRAY

Your thermic fuel is divided into 5 food groups for convenient use: (1) Protein, (2) Dairy, (3) Starches, (4) Vegetables, and (5) Fruit.

The foods in each group were rated and calculated to provide all the nutrients you need daily. In addition, serving sizes were computed to design your Daily Diet Tray. This Daily Tray is your complete food plan or blueprint for eating the right foods in the right amounts for a nutritionally balanced 1,000-calorie fat-burning diet.

Each day, you will eat:

- 2 servings protein.
- 2 servings dairy.
- 4 servings starches.
- 4 servings vegetables.
- 3 servings fruit.

YOUR DAILY DIET HOTPLATES

How you eat your food is just as important as what you are eating to achieve a better thermic burn.

To get the best thermic effect from your Daily Tray, you want to keep your thermic foods coming, to keep your thermic response burning at high power.

You want to turn on your thermic switch in the morning and keep it as hot as you can until it's time for you to turn in for the evening. Like a fire in a cold room, you want to keep the fire stoked to keep the heat constant.

To do that, you are going to eat your calories in a certain way, on three Daily Diet *Hotplates*.

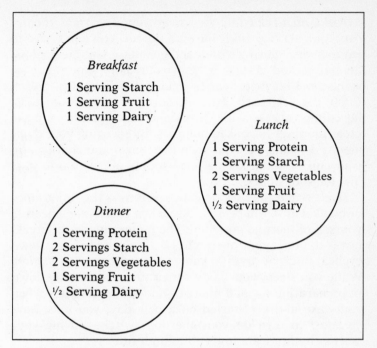

Note: Carbohydrates are all foods except protein and fat.

A PERFECT THERMIC DAY

- Eat at least 3 meals a day, never skipping breakfast.
- Eat at least 2 carbohydrates for breakfast.
- *No fat before noon.* Since fat has the lowest thermic response, you don't want to add your fat until your higher level of physical activity can offset that fat intake.
- Double your carbohydrates at lunch, with protein for muscle preservation.
- Keep your fires going with most of your carbohydrates at dinner, and protein for muscle protection.

By dividing your fuel this way, you will get the best overall thermic effect from your daily diet.

A note about calcium: We spread your 2 servings of dairy over 3 meals. We did it for *meal appeal.* You don't need to eat too "dry" during a diet, and one place you can get low-fat sauces and gravies is from your dairy group. For instance, low-fat yogurt can be made into a delightful "Peach Crisp" dessert (see the Thermic Burn Recipes section). Low-fat cottage cheese with chives and other garnishes make great toppings for baked potatoes. By splitting your dairy among 3 meals, you can keep the charm and charisma in your cuisine—and keep a good supply of calcium in your diet for your bones.

Don't skip breakfast! We can't overstress the importance of breakfast. If you're not a breakfast eater, *stop* cheating yourself of thermic potential. The major purpose of breakfast is to break your overnight fast. Your body has its own cyclical internal rhythm, known as your *circadian rhythm.* While you sleep, your body's thermostat turns way down in preparation for 6–8 hours of no food or activity. When you wake and get started on a new day, you *must have breakfast* to turn on your thermic switch, moving your body's rhythm from low ebb to high tide.

Meal planning made easy: The distribution of your foods was also made with variety in mind, to help you fix interesting meals. We distributed your fruit and dairy evenly and together, so they can be eaten in combination as a dessert or mixed with your other foods for a change of pace. For instance, chicken with spicy applesauce on the side can be used as a low-fat substitute for sweet and sour sauce.

Snacks: If you need a snack during the day, you can use one or two of your portions from lunch or dinner, but then don't eat them again. *Never* get your snacks from your breakfast hotplate.

YOUR FAT-TO-MUSCLE FOOD LISTS

Your Daily Diet Hotplates will carry you through the entire term of your diet. We provide two different Thermic Food

Lists (Burn 1 and Burn 2), with a different fat maximum to use for each phase of your diet. From these lists, you will choose the foods you need to match your Daily Hotplates for great meals.

To develop your Thermic Food Lists, we analyzed over 1,000 foods, rating the ones that would work the best for you. We narrowed the range of your thermic fuel, choosing foods with the most power for the fewest calories. We censored some of the high-fat problem foods, and limited your portions of medium-fat foods, to teach you a simple fact about fat: It's not that you can't have fat, but when you do, you have to limit your portions. Through the diet, you will be portioning your fats automatically and you'll learn as you go along. When you're comfortable eating fat in smaller portions, you've got the "secret" for staying low-fat for life. By the end of your diet, you'll *need* less fat and feel better eating less fat.

We're proud of our built-in plan of attack against fat. We think you'll like it too. You won't have to worry about breaking the bad habit of eating fat. You'll learn as you move through your diet. In addition, you'll have a backup plan in Burn 1 and Burn 2 that you can rely on in case you find yourself eating more fat at maintenance.

For these reasons, your Fat-to-Muscle Diet is even more than a system for high-powered burning. It's an educational system for trouble-free learning.

You've got the power on your side to break your fat habit for life. You can stand up to it. You can beat fat.

FIVE

THE BURN 1 AND BURN 2 DIETS

BURN 1

This is the first phase of your Fat-to-Muscle Diet. Study the following Thermic Food Lists and read Creating Meal Menus to find out how to use the foods to create a perfect thermic day.

Burn 1

Breakfast
1 Serving Starch
1 Serving Fruit
1 Serving Dairy

Lunch
1 Serving Protein
1 Serving Starch
2 Servings Vegetables
1 Serving Fruit
½ Serving Dairy

Dinner
1 Serving Protein
2 Servings Starch
2 Servings Vegetables
1 Serving Fruit
½ Serving Dairy

Guidelines
- Select foods and servings that complete each meal Hotplate.
- Limit alcohol to *no more* than 2 drinks per week.
- Do not eliminate any foods.
- Closely follow the portions listed.
- Limit choice from Optional List to 1 per day.

Protein		Dairy		Starches		Vegetables		Fruit	
Food	Serv.	Food	Serv.	Food	Serv.	Food	Serv.	Food	Serv.
Bass	3 oz	Buttermilk	1 c	Bagel, (5" dia.)	½	Alfalfa sprouts	2 oz	Apple, small	1
Beef, round, no fat	3 oz	Cottage cheese, low-fat	⅔ c	Bread, all sliced	1 sl	Artichoke hearts	4	Apple butter	1 tbsp
Black beans	⅔ c	Low-fat milk	½ c	Bread sticks	2	Asparagus spears	8	Apple juice	3 oz
Bluefish	3 oz	Skim milk	½ c	Bulgur, cooked	1 cup	Bamboo shoots	½ c	Applesauce	½ c
Chicken, no skin	3 oz	Yogurt, plain, low-fat	1 cup	Cereal, cooked	1 cup	Beans, green/ wax	½ c	Apricot, fresh	1
Clams	15 or	Yogurt, va-nilla/fruit, low-fat	½ c	Cereal, dry	1 c or	Bean sprouts	1 c	Apricot halves	4
Cod	3 oz					Beets	1 oz	Apricot nectar	2 oz
Crabmeat	3 oz							Banana	½
								Blueberries	½ c
								Cantaloupe	¼
								Cherries	½ c

Protein		Dairy		Starches		Vegetables		Fruit	
Food	*Serv.*	*Food*	*Serv.*	*Food*	*Serv.*	*Food*	*Serv.*	*Food*	*Serv.*
Egg, whites only	2			Corn on cob	1/2	Broccoli	1/2	Cranberry juice	1/2
Flounder	3 oz			Corn kernels	1/2 c	Brussels sprouts	1/2 c	Cranberry sauce	2 oz
Garbanzos (chick peas)	1/2 c			Crackers, melba	7	Cabbage	1 c	Dates	1/4 c
Great northern beans	2/3 c			Crackers, oyster	20	Carrots	1/2 c	Figs	2
Haddock	3 oz			Crackers, rice cake	2	Cauliflower	1 c	Fruit cocktail	1
Halibut	3 oz			Macaroni, cooked	1/2 c	Celery	1 c	Grapefruit	1/2 c
Kidney beans	2/3 c			Parsnips	1/2 c	Cucumber, small	1	Grapefruit juice	1/2
Lentils	2/3 c			Peas, green	1/2 c	Greens	1/2 c	Grapes	4 oz
Lobster	3 oz			Pita bread	1/2	Eggplant	1 c	Honeydew melon	10
Mackerel	3 oz			Potato, baked	1/2	Lettuce	2 c	Kiwi	1/8
Oysters	10 or 1 c			Popcorn, no oil	3 c	Mushrooms	1 c	Lemon	1
Rockfish	3 oz			Rice, any kind, cooked	1/2 c	Okra	1 c	Lime	2
Scallops	3 oz			Roll, dinner	1	Onion	1/2 c	Mango	1/2
Shrimp	20 or 3 oz			Roll, hard	1/2	Pepper, sweet	1 c	Orange	1
Sole	3 oz			Roll, soft (bun)	1/2	Snow peas	1 c	Orange juice	4 oz
Swordfish	3 oz					Spinach	1 c	Papaya	1 c
Tuna, in water	3 oz					Squash, summer	1 c	Peach, fresh	1
						Tomato	1	Peach, halves	2

Protein		Protein		Starches		Vegetables		Fruit	
Food	Serv.	Food	Serv.	Food	Serv.	Food	Serv.	Food	Serv.
Turkey, no skin	3 oz	Green pea (milk)	1 c	Spaghetti, noodles	½ c	Tomato, canned	½ c	Pear, fresh	½
Venison	3 oz	Split pea (ready)	1 c	Squash, winter	⅔ c	Tomato juice	1 c	Pear, halves	2
Soups (canned):		Turkey chunk (ready)	1 c	Tortilla (6" dia.)	1	Zucchini	1 c	Persimmon	1
Black bean (water)	1 c			Turnips	1 c			Pineapple	½ c
Beef chunk (ready)	1 c			Soups (canned):				Pineapple juice	4 oz
Chicken and rice (ready)	1 c			Broth	1 c			Plum	1
Chicken and vegetable (ready)	1 c			Chicken and vegetable	1 c			Prunes	2
Manhattan clam chowder	1 c			Consommé	1 c			Prune juice	2 oz
Crab (ready)	1 c			Vegetable	1 c			Raisins	2 tbsp
Lentil with ham (ready)	1 c							Raspberries	½ c
Minestrone (ready)	1 c							Strawberries	1 c
								Watermelon	1 c

Optional

Food	Serv.	Food	Serv.
Angelfood cake	1 piece	Fruit juice pop	1
Honey	1 tbsp	Popsicle	1
Jelly/jam	1 tbsp	Sherbet	½ c

CREATING MEAL MENUS

Matching your food choices to your Hotplates: To use the Fat-to-Muscle Diet, you simply choose your foods from each food group on the Burn 1 Food Sheets and match them to the servings required for each day.

Following is a sample day that shows you how flexible and varied the diet can be. Now try creating your own meals.

Your Meal		Breakfast	
	Day 1	Day 2	Day 3
(1 serving starch)	1 c cereal	½ bagel	½ English muffin
(1 serving dairy)	1 c skim milk	½ c low-fat milk	1 c plain yogurt
(1 serving fruit)	½ banana	¼ cantaloupe	2 peach halves*
(1 serving optional)		1 tsp jelly	

*Fruit and dairy can be combined for fabulous desserts (see recipes).

Your Meal		Lunch	
	Day 1	Day 2	Day 3
	Cold pasta salad	Stuffed pita pocket	Chicken sandwich tortilla
(1 serving protein)	3 oz crabmeat	3 oz tuna, in water	3 oz chicken
(1 serving starch)	½ c macaroni, cooked	½ pita pocket	1 tortilla
(1 serving vegetable)	½ c green pepper*	½ c onions*	1 cucumber, speared
	½ tomato*	½ tomato*	
(1 serving vegetable)	½ c snow peas*	1 c lettuce*	¼ c carrots, shredded*
	½ mushrooms*	½ c celery*	½ c celery, chopped*
(½ serving dairy)	½ c plain yogurt with mixed herbs	½ c skim milk	¼ c vanilla yogurt†
(1 serving fruit)	¼ cantaloupe	1 orange	1 c strawberries

*Half servings of food can be added together to make 1 serving.
†Fruit and dairy can be combined for fabulous desserts (see recipes).

| | Dinner | | |
Your Meal	Day 1	Day 2	Day 3
(1 serving protein)	3 oz swordfish, baked	3 oz lean round beef	3 oz turkey, roasted
(2 serving starch)	1 baked potato*	1 corn on cob*	1 dinner roll 1 c vegetable soup
(2 servings vegetables)	1 c broccoli*	1 large salad‡	½ c carrots 1 small salad‡
(1 serving fruit)	1 plum	1 c blueberries	½ c fruit cocktail
(½ serving daily)	¼ c low-fat cottage cheese with chives (for potato)†	½ c plain yogurt† (mix with fruit)	½ c skim milk†

*Double portions equal 2 servings.

†Use half portions for half servings.

‡Small mixed salads equal 1 serving vegetables; large mixed salads equal 2 servings vegetables.

Are you getting the idea? Your three Hotplates give you the format to make fabulous meals. Eat fancy or plain. Toss salads with small portions of many vegetables. You can eat like royalty on a low-fat diet with plenty of carbohydrates and protein to achieve thermic burn.

Eat all of the servings, no more or less. Never eat less! Less is not better. Less is not nutritious. You will not lose fat faster with less. Never eat less!

Check our recipe collection for some mouth-watering recipes you can plug into your day, and eat low-fat gourmet the easy way.

MENUS AND RECIPES: GOURMET DINING ON THE FAT-TO-MUSCLE DIET

We want you to succeed. That means eating thermically even if you don't have time to select your foods and work them into three daily meals. So we went a step further with your program. Paul Gizara, who received his culinary training from the Culinary Institute of America, developed mouth-watering recipes for both phases of your Fat-to-Muscle Diet— Burn 1 and Burn 2. We planned them into daily menus to meet your Hotplate requirements and to satisfy your sense of taste.

When you're in a hurry, use the menus to make your day.

To insure that you don't mix up your daily portions, when you use a menu, use *the whole day*. Don't try to take a lunch from the menus and balance the rest of the day in your head. You might underestimate or overestimate your portions. *Use the whole day when you use a menu instead of the food plan.*

As an extra added attraction, we included recipes for gourmet dining on a thermic diet. You can pull out a recipe and use it as part of your daily plan, because we indicated the number of servings the recipe represents. Check the appendix for 4 full weeks of Burn 1 and Burn 2 menus, plus mouth-watering recipes.

Your Thermic Diet Options: You could use the menus to take you through your entire program, following the Thermic Burn Diet exclusively by menus. But we'd like you to get used to choosing and using your own foods. That's the way you'll learn how to find fat, figure it, and fight it. That's how you will learn to eat thermically, and that will carry you through life. But you do have the option of no-think thermogenesis.

As you can see, we've thought of everything! And our chef made everything sing. You can eat like royalty when you're eating thermically.

BURN 2

You get to choose a litte more fat from a new *fat food group* and your selection of food is expanded to include higher-fat food choices.

Plan your menus just as you did during Burn 1, using the Burn 2 Hotplates listed on your Burn 2 food lists.

Notice! You are going to increase the intensity of your exercise to back up this boost in food fat and food choices. Refer to your Diet Calendar for details. This will keep you on track for burning fat straight through to the end of your diet.

Burn 2

Breakfast	Lunch	Dinner
1 Serving Starch	1 Serving Protein	1 Serving Protein
1 Serving Fruit	1 Serving Starch	2 Servings Starch
1 Serving Dairy	2 Servings Vegetables	2 Servings Vegetables
	1 Serving Fruit	1 Serving Fruit
	½ Serving Dairy	½ Serving Dairy
	1 Serving Fat*	

Guidelines

- Select foods and servings that complete each meal Hotplate.
- Limit alcohol to *no more than* 2 drinks per week.
- Do not eliminate any foods.
- Closely follow the portions listed.
- Limit choice from Optional List to 1 per day.

Protein

Food	Serv.
Bass	3 oz
Beef, round, no fat	3 oz
Black beans	⅔ c
Bluefish	3 oz
Chicken, no skin	3 oz
Clams	15 or 3 oz
Cod	3 oz
Crabmeat	3 oz
Egg, whites only	2

Dairy

Food	Serv.
Buttermilk	1 c
Cottage cheese, low-fat	½ c
Low-fat milk	½ c
Skim milk	1 cup
Yogurt, plain, low-fat	1 cup
Yogurt, vanilla/fruit, low-fat	½ c

Starches

Food	Serv.
Bagel, (5" dia.)	½
Bread, all sliced	1 sl
Bread sticks	2
Bulgur, cooked	½ c
Cereal, cooked	1 cup
Cereal, dry	1 c or 1 oz
Corn on cob	½
Corn kernels	½ c

Vegetables

Food	Serv.
Alfalfa sprouts	2 oz
Artichoke hearts	4
Asparagus spears	8
Bamboo shoots	½ c
Beans, green/wax	1 c
Bean sprouts	½ c
Beets	½ c
Broccoli	½

Fruit

Food	Serv.
Apple, small	1
Apple butter	1 tbsp
Apple juice	3 oz
Applesauce	½ c
Apricot, fresh	1
Apricot halves	4
Apricot nectar	2 oz
Banana	½
Blueberries	½ c
Cantaloupe	¼
Cherries	½ c
Cranberry juice	2 oz

Protein		Dairy		Starches		Vegetables		Fruit	
Food	Serv.	Food	Serv.	Food	Serv.	Food	Serv.	Food	Serv.
Flounder	3 oz			Crackers, melba	7	Brussels sprouts	½ c	Cranberry sauce	¼ c
Garbanzos (chick peas)	½ c			Crackers, oyster	20	Cabbage	1 c	Dates	2
Great northern beans	⅔ c			Crackers, rice cake	2	Carrots	½ c	Figs	1
Haddock	3 oz			Macaroni, cooked	½ c	Cauliflower	1 c	Fruit cocktail	½ c
Halibut	3 oz			Parsnips	½ c	Celery	1 c	Grapefruit	½
Kidney beans	⅔ c			Peas, green	½ c	Cucumber, small	1	Grapefruit juice	4 oz
Lentils	⅔ c			Pita bread	½	Greens	½ c	Grapes	10
Lobster	3 oz			Potato, baked	½	Eggplant	1 c	Honeydew melon	⅛
Mackerel	3 oz			Popcorn, no oil	3 c	Lettuce	2 c	Kiwi	1
Oysters	10 or 1 c			Rice, any kind, cooked	½ c	Mushrooms	1 c	Lemon	2
Rockfish	3 oz			Roll, dinner	1	Okra	1 c	Lime	2
Scallops	3 oz			Roll, hard	½	Onion	½ c	Mango	½
Shrimp	20 or 3 oz			Roll, soft (bun)	½	Pepper, sweet	1 c	Orange	1
Sole	3 oz			Spaghetti, noodles	½ c	Snow peas	1 c	Orange juice	4 oz
Swordfish	3 oz			Squash, winter	⅔ c	Spinach	1 c	Papaya	1 c
Tuna, in water	3 oz					Squash, summer	1 c	Peach, fresh	1
Turkey, no skin	3 oz					Tomato	1	Peach, halves	2
Venison	3 oz					Tomato, canned	½ c	Pear, fresh	½
						Tomato juice	1 c	Pear, halves	2
						Zucchini	1 c	Persimmon	1

Protein		Dairy		Starches		Vegetables		Fruit	
Food	Serv.	Food	Serv.	Food	Serv.	Food	Serv.	Food	Serv.
Soups (canned):				Tortilla (6" dia.)	1			Pineapple	½ c
Black bean (water)	1 c			Turnips	1 c			Pineapple juice	4 oz
Beef chunk (ready)	1 c			Soups (canned):				Plum	1
Chicken and rice (ready)	1 c			Broth	1 c			Prunes	2
Chicken and vegetable (ready)	1 c			Chicken and vegetable	1 c			Prune juice	2 oz
Manhattan clam chowder	1 c			Consommé	1 c			Raisins	2 tbsp
Crab (ready)	1 c			Vegetable	1 c			Raspberries	½ c
Lentil with ham (ready)	1 c			Corn bread	1 sl			Strawberries	1 c
Minestrone (ready)	1 c			Crackers, graham	1			Watermelon	1 c
Green pea (milk)	1 c			Crackers, saltines	5				
Split pea (ready)	1 c			Granola cereal	1 oz				
Turkey chunk (ready)	1 c			Pancakes (6" dia.)	1				
				Roll, ready to eat	1				
				Taco shell	1				
				Waffle	1				
				Wheat germ	1 tbsp				

Protein		Fats		Starches	
Food	*Serv.*	*Food*	*Serv.*	*Food*	*Serv.*
Anchovy	10	Almonds	½ oz	*Soups* (canned):	
Baked beans	⅓ c	Avocado	⅛	Beef boullion	1 c
Beef:		Bacon	2 sl	Beef noodle (water)	1 c
Chuck, no fat	2 oz	Butter	1 tsp	Chicken broth (water)	1 c
Ground (10%)	2 oz	Cashews	½ oz	Chicken gumbo (water)	1 c
Loin	2 oz	Coconut	¼ c	Chicken noodle (water)	1 c
Round, with fat	2 oz	Cream cheese	1 tbsp	Chicken rice (water)	1 c
Rump, no fat	2 oz	Cream, sour	1 tbsp	Chicken vegetable	
Steak, no fat	2 oz	Cream, whip	1 tbsp	(water)	1 c
Bologna, Lebanon	2 oz	*Gravies:*		Onion (water)	1 c
Canadian bacon	2 oz	Au jus	⅓ c	Scotch broth (water)	1 c
Caviar	2 oz	Beef, canned	½ c	Tomato bisque (milk)	1 c
Chicken:		Chicken, canned	¼ c	Tomato (milk)	1 c
with skin	2 oz	Mushroom, canned	¼ c	Tomato rice (water)	1 c
Drumstick	1	Lard	1 tbsp	Turkey noodle (water)	1 c
Roll	2 oz	Margarine	1 tsp	Vegetable chunk	
Salad	⅓ c	Mayonnaise	1 tbsp	(ready)	1 c
Wing	1	Olives	10	Vegetable (water)	1 c
Crab, deviled	¼ c	Peanuts	½ oz	Vegetable beef (water)	1 c
Fish cakes	1	Pecans	½ oz		
Ham, baked	2 oz	Pistachios	½ oz		
Ham, boiled	2 oz	Salad dressings	1 tbsp		

Protein		Fats		Optional	
Food	Serv.	Food	Serv.	Food	Serv.
Herring, pickled	2 oz	*Sauces:*		Angelfood cake	1 piece
Lamb, trimmed	2 oz	Béarnaise	⅛ c	Honey	1 tbsp
Liver, calf	2 oz	Cheese	¼ c	Jelly/jam	1 tbsp
Pork, loin/chops, no fat	2 oz	Curry	¼ c	Fruit juice pop	1
Salmon	2 oz	Hollandaise	¼ c	Popsicle	1
Tofu	4 oz	Stroganoff	¼ c	Sherbet	½ c
Turkey roll	2 oz	Tartar	1 tbsp		
Veal	2 oz	White	¼ c		
		Sesame seeds	1 tbsp		
		Sunflower seeds	¼ c		
		Walnuts	½ oz		

SIX

STARTING YOUR DIET

CHOOSING YOUR GOAL

Body Status

	Body Status	*Percent Body Fat*	*Percent Muscle*
Women	Very-Low-Fat-Lean	10–17%	90–83%
	Low-Fat-Slim	17–22	83–78
	Average-Fat-Ideal	22–25	78–75
	Above-Average-Trouble	25–29	75–71
Men	Very-Low-Fat-Lean	7–10%	93–90%
	Low-Fat-Slim	10–15	90–85
	Average-Fat-Ideal	15–18	85–82
	Above-Average-Trouble	18–10	82–80

Choose your fat-to-muscle goal from the Body Status Chart and follow the recommended diet program for that goal. The Fat-to-Muscle Diet was designed in two phases to adapt to various goals.

- Burn 1: This is the strictest fat-cutting part of the program, designed to break your addiction to fat. The fat maximum is 15–18 percent of your total calories, which means that the fats you are eating are hidden fats.

• Burn 2:   This phase introduces a *fat* category into your food system and you are allowed to choose one extra fat. The fat maximum is 20–25 percent of your calories. This phase is a gradual transition from Burn 1 and you must use it for at least one week before the end of your diet.

MATCHING YOUR DIET TO YOUR GOAL

• Low-Fat-Slim (Aggressive Goal):

Follow Burn 1 until you reach your satisfied size. Then use 2 weeks of Burn 2 to ease you back into eating fat. Follow the exercise schedule planned into your Diet Calendar.

• Average-Fat-Ideal (Recommended Goal):

Follow Burn 1 for two weeks and move on to Burn 2 until you reach a weight you are satisfied with. If you hit trouble spots and start eating more fat, go back to Burn 1 and use it as a booster for a week. Follow the exercise schedule in your Diet Calendar.

• Above-Average-Trouble:

This is a step goal for people who start out very high-fat obese. Follow Burn 1 for two weeks, then Burn 2 for two weeks, then go back and repeat until you reach your satisfied size. The more fat you have, the longer your diet will last. This program of alternating diets will allow you enough variety to continue the program over the long term. If you find that you feel strong and confident after a few cycles and don't need more food variety and fat, stay on Burn 1 and go for it with gusto! Follow the exercise schedule in your Diet Calendar but use *only brisk walking* for exercise, unless you have medical approval to move on to the higher-intensity aerobics. Generally, people can handle higher-intensity exercise when they are within 30 pounds of their goal. *Remember:* The heavier you are, the more you need exercise. Don't think for a minute that you can skip exercise. Clock your time, and start at your own pace. Check with your physician first if you have any questions or doubts. You might take longer to get to your goal, but you'll have twice as much to celebrate when you get there.

• Very-Low-Fat-Lean (Are you sure?): This is a goal usually achieved only by highly trained athletes. If you are already fit, but have a little extra fat, and wish to achieve a leaner physique, follow Burn 1 for a low-fat foundation but increase your complex carbohydrates to satisfy your increased calorie needs from your intensive training efforts. Consult an exercise physiologist for specific guidelines

on building and training. A note
of caution: Make sure your desire to be very lean doesn't su-
percede your ability to achieve
top performance. Some athletes, even runners, perform best
at a slightly higher percentage
of body fat.

Now you're ready to start the Fat-to-Muscle Diet! Open
your calendar and follow along until you reach your ideal
goal.

SEVEN

YOUR FAT-TO-MUSCLE CALENDAR

Day by day, you are going to reduce your fat, increase your muscle, and increase your thermic response. Day by day, you will fine-tune your metabolism by eating right, exercising right, and changing habits that have harmed you into habits that will improve your life.

One of the main reasons diets fail (outside of muscle loss) is that dieters can't stick to them. This sounds like a simple issue, but it involves a host of complicated behavioral problems that go back to the habits that cause fat gain in the first place.

Over the years, the diet business has boomed, and hundreds of diets have come and gone, but most have served only to *take away* your better eating habits and behavior, replacing them with crazy food combinations, magic pills, formulas, and fads that make you think there's some secret road to fitness. What this does behaviorally is give control of your life to something outside yourself.

Developing control over your life means knowing what to eat, how to eat, how to exercise, what choices to make, how to manage stress, how to cope with your diet, and how to fit it into your schedule. How to succeed in taking charge of your life. That's a lot to juggle in an already busy life.

Your Fat-to-Muscle Calendar will give you back control

over your eating, exercise, and habits. You will regain the good habits you lost somewhere along the line and learn several new techniques to keep you on the success track.

Your calendar carefully builds a perfect diet month for you, giving you control over your diet in an easy-to-use, follow-along style. Even if you simply follow it without thinking, a pattern is being introduced into your daily life, and that pattern will teach you by itself. The keys to fitness are in *taking charge*, and as you watch your days taking on a fitness pattern, the sense of control will flow over into the other areas of your life.

You've probably heard the old adage: When you have your health, you have everything. That's true, but it means more than having your health like a gift or a blessing. It means *taking it*. Taking charge of your life.

YOUR FAT-TO-MUSCLE CALENDAR is designed for your success. It includes a complete program for improving your lifestyle, with a thermic diet to burn fat, aerobic exercise to raise your muscle status, pre-planning behavior to start you on the success track, and special boosters to ward off stress. You are getting THE BIG THREE built right in— DIET, EXERCISE, AND BEHAVIOR MODIFICATION FOR LIFESTYLE IMPROVEMENT. Check your goal and follow the recommended program.

> LOW-FAT-SLIM: Follow Burn 1 to satisfied size. Follow up with two weeks of Burn 2.
>
> AVERAGE-FAT-IDEAL: Follow Burn 1 for two weeks. Take Burn 2 to your satisfied size. Trouble spots? Use Burn 1 as a one-week booster.
>
> ABOVE-AVERAGE, STEP GOAL: Follow Burn 1 for two weeks. Switch to Burn 2 for two weeks. Go back and repeat until you reach your satisfied size.

Check the boxes each day you meet the goals. If you don't meet the goal, don't check the box. At the end of each week, go back and reassess your problem areas—the ones you didn't check. Keep an eye on meeting all of the goals the next week.

Fat-to-Muscle Calendar

3 PREPREPARATION DAYS

	Day 1	Day 2	Day 3
	EAT NORMALLY □ Record Intake Read: □ "Setting Yourself Up Right" □ "Figuring Degree of Fat Trouble" □ "Ideal Body *What?*" □ "Your Scale" □ "Water . . ."	EAT NORMALLY □ Record Intake Read: □ "Gaining Mental Muscle." □ "Creating Your Diet Environment" □ "Thermic Action" chapter	EAT NORMALLY □ Record and Tally □ Study Burn 1 Diet and food lists Read: □ "Creating Meal Menus" □ Work out sample menus □ Make shopping list, □ Get foods! Get ready!

USE THE BOXES TO CHECK OFF COMPLETION OF DAY'S REQUIREMENTS

START BURN 1					
□ Eat Hotplates □ Exercise* □ 8 Gl Liquid □ Read "Eating low-fat"	□ Eat Hotplates □ 8 Gl Liquid □ Read "Why you eat . . ."	□ Eat Hotplates □ Exercise □ 8 Gl Liquid □ Read "Emergency Thermic Boosters"	□ Eat Hotplates □ 8 Gl Liquid	□ Eat Hotplates □ Exercise □ 8 Gl Liquid □ Read "Rewards"	□ Eat Hotplates □ 8 Gl Liquid □ Reward! □ Get foods!

CONT. BURN 1 □ Eat Hotplates □ Exercise □ 8 Gl Liquid	□ Eat Hotplates □ Exercise □ 8 Gl Liquid	□ Eat Hotplates □ 8 Gl Liquid □ Read "Relief" and Practice	□ Eat Hotplates □ 8 Gl Liquid	□ Hotplate □ Exercise □ Liquid Are you moving on to Burn 2?†	□ Eat Hotplates □ 8 Gl Liquid □ Reward! □ Get foods!
BURN 2 □ Eat Hotplates □ Exercise □ 8 Gl Liquid □ Read "Emergency Thermic Boosters" □ Remeasure yourself	□ Eat Hotplates □ Exercise □ 8 Gl Liquid	□ Eat Hotplates □ 8 Gl Liquid □ Do "Relief" □ Not overeating fat	□ Eat Hotplates □ Exercise □ 8 Gl Liquid	□ Eat Hotplates □ 8 Gl Liquid □ Do "Relief"	□ Eat Hotplates □ Exercise □ 8 Gl Liquid □ Reward! □ Get foods
□ Eat Hotplates □ Exercise □ 8 Gl Liquid □ Read "Facing Up to Stress" and Practice	□ Eat Hotplates □ Exercise □ 8 Gl Liquid	□ Eat Hotplates □ 8 Gl Liquid □ Do "Relief" □ Not overeating fat	□ Eat Hotplates □ Exercise □ 8 Gl Liquid	□ Eat Hotplates □ 8 Gl Liquid □ Do "Relief"	□ Eat Hotplates □ Exercise □ 8 Gl Liquid □ Reward! □ Get foods! end?‡ □ Read Maintenance chapter

*Exercise. You can take this any days of the week that are convenient. In Burn 1—at least 3 days; in Burn 2—at least 4 days.
†Study Burn 2 thermic food list. Make sample menu. Make shopping list. Follow this on the last week you are on Burn 1.
‡CONGRATULATIONS!!!
IF YOU BREAK YOUR DIET, READ: HOW TO HANDLE A DIET BREAKDOWN.

SETTING YOURSELF UP RIGHT

The first 3 days of your program are dedicated to preprep-aration. *This is a vital step in your Fat-to-Muscle program.* Don't skip prepreparation, thinking you can jump right into the diet and do all your calculations then. The preprepa-ration days are a very important behavior modification technique. When you come into a diet without the proper preparation, too often you have to keep backtracking to pick up missing pieces. Setting yourself up right means setting yourself up for success.

For the first 3 days of your program, *eat normally. Don't start dieting yet!*

During these 3 days, you will be recording what you eat and figuring the degree of fat trouble in your food.

Dieting is *stress.* You want to remove as many questions as possible before you move into the fat loss phase.

Don't skip these 3 days. Later, you'll realize the benefits in success.

FIGURING DEGREE OF FAT TROUBLE

During the first 3 days, you are going to *fat scan* what you eat. In a sense, you are going to act as your personal diet-itian.

Set aside a notebook to be used exclusively for your Fat-to-Muscle Diet. Include your meals, foods eaten, and the approximate portion size. Don't forget those calorie-packed condiments such as pats of butter and cream in your coffee.

Write down everything you eat and drink for 3 days. List all of the snacks and nibbles that you eat in a typical day, including soft drinks. Don't leave it for your mind to re-member—your mind has better things to do.

Keep track of 3 days, and if you can, include a weekend day. Have fun with this. Think of yourself as a detective on an important case, staking out fat for a big reward.

Eat normally. Don't start cutting fat yet. Don't try to eat

less so your record looks better. Don't fool yourself. No one is going to use these records but you. If you eat 2 potato chips, list them. Be realistic and measure your portions without underestimating them. Don't forget alcohol. Don't forget snacks—five nibbled nuts are 4 grams of fat. A handful of nuts are 20 grams. List them.

- At the end of each day, tally the total calories and fat grams that you ate, using the Fat Gram Counter at the end of this book. If you can't find a brand name food in our counter, use the generic food. If your food is not listed, check the food label for fat content and calories.
- At the end of the third day, total the calories and fat grams for the 3 days, and divide by 3 to get a 3-day average.
- To figure the average percentage of fat in your diet, multiply your average 3-day total of fat grams by 9 (calories per gram of fat). Then divide that number by your average total calories for the 3 days. This will give you the percent of your total calories that is fat.
- Example: Average total calories for 3 days = 2000 calories
  Average total fat grams for 3 days = 89 grams
  89 grams fat × 9 (cals per gram) = 801 calories
  801 calories from fat ÷ 2,000 total cals = 40% cals as fat.

Your daily diet should not contain more than 25 percent of its total calories as fat—or more than 50–55 grams per day, as an upper limit.

Below is a sample of an average American daily diet. On first glance it doesn't look too threatening, but closer inspection will reveal that the fat maxed over the ceiling for anyone, with a daily fat intake of 136 grams.

	Daily Fat Diary	Fat Grams
Breakfast:	Cheese omelet	26
	2 slices bacon	8
	Toast with butter	4
	Coffee with cream	2
	Orange juice	0
Lunch:	Tuna salad sandwich (with mayo)	11
	French fries	15
	Coffee with cream	2
	Fruit	0
Dinner:	6-oz steak	18
	Baked potato with sour cream	6
	Broccoli with butter	4
	Bread with butter	8
	Salad with dressing	24
Snack:	Ice cream	8
	Total fat grams:	136

EIGHT

THERMIC ACTION: YOUR EXERCISE HOTLIST

Burn 1: Choose 1 of the following aerobic exercises and work out for 30 minutes, 3 days per week or every other day. You can vary your exercise selections within each week. Begin your exercise on the *first* day you start dieting.

Burn 2: Choose 1 or a combination of the following exercises and work out for 30 minutes, 4 days per week.

- *Action aerobics:* brisk walking, swimming, jogging, aerobic dance.
- *Marvelous machines:* rowing machine, rebounding, stationary bicycle, treadmill, Nordic track.
- *Skill sport aerobics:* tennis, racquetball, squash, handball, skiing, basketball, volleyball.

Note: If you start your diet as high-fat obese, choose *only* brisk walking for the first few weeks, and get your doctor's approval to begin more strenuous workouts. Rule of Thumb: 30 pounds from your ideal weight is a safe range for more vigorous exercise.

Before You Start: Learn to take your target heart rate. Remember to warm up and cool down, in addition to your aerobic exercise. Brisk walking is the only exercise that acts as its own warm-up and cool-down.

ACTION AEROBICS

Brisk Walking

Walk briskly but work up to a good pace slowly.

Degree of Difficulty: Low.

Benefits:
- Excellent cardiovascular workout.
- Low-intensity exercise where more time is spent at a less strenuous level.
- Convenient: no special equipment necessary, except good shoes; easy to schedule into your day.
- No special skills required.
- Excellent stress manager.
- Can be enjoyed alone or with friends.
- Minimal injury compared to jogging.
- Great for lunchtime break.
- High degree of peer support.
- Fun for beginners and seasoned exercisers.
- Pace easily adapted.
- Easily transferred to indoor track or mall for inclement weather.
- Good grounder for people who live and work in high-rise apartments.

Walking develops muscle tone, strength, endurance, flexibility, and agility. Joggers say that running puts them in touch with their bodies, but walking goes one step further— it gives you time and space to reflect on yourself and your environment. The visual stimulation of walking is less stressful than jogging, with fast-forward films running across your eyes. You can enjoy nature or your city, noticing things that might otherwise have passed you by.

Guidelines:
- In the beginning, duration is more important than distance.
- Begin with modest distances and gradually increase your speed as walking becomes more comfortable.

- Swing your arms rhythmically and try to breathe deeply.
- Strike the longest stride that is comfortable for you.
- Keep your momentum steady and think about being light, putting less weight on your feet.
- Wear light, comfortable clothes and shoes that don't slip or rub.

Walking Incentives:
- Adopt a dog.
- Walk with a friend.
- In bad weather, walk a mall or an indoor track at a school or gym.
- Make a list of creative reasons to walk.
- *Plan* your walk into your day!

Swimming

Degree of Difficulty: Low–High (depending on speed and stroke).

Benefits:
- Excellent cardiovascular training.
- Good calorie-burning exercise.
- No injury to joints.
- Works upper and lower body.
- Improves range of arm motion.
- Pools available at most community centers.
- Good exercise to combine with other activities.

Guidelines:
- Purchase a comfortable swimming suit and goggles to protect eyes.
- Scout local community centers and colleges for available pools and swimming hours.
- Ask about length of a pool and number of laps (pool lengths) that equal a mile. Use this as a challenge for gradually increasing your distance.

- Find a convenient time when crowds are light, allowing you full pool length for working out.
- Combine stroke styles for variety (i.e., crawl, breast stroke, back stroke, side stroke, butterfly—if you can do this difficult stroke).
- Combine with another activity of weight-bearing nature (such as brisk walking) to increase calcium absorption in bones for building skeletal strength.

Jogging

Degree of Difficulty: Medium–High.

Benefits:
- Excellent cardiovascular training.
- Excellent calorie-burning activity.
- Convenient: requires only the time to get dressed, warm up, and go.
- Able to enjoy the fresh outdoors, altering your path for variety.
- Easily transferred to an indoor track.
- High degree of peer support.

Guidelines:
- Jogging should not be an exercise choice if you are more than 30 pounds over your goal weight.
- A walk-jog pattern can be incorporated (walk 5 minutes, jog 2 minutes, for example) as you gradually improve your level of fitness.
- Make sure you have very supportive running shoes and proper attire for the climate.
- Stop jogging (and walk) if you experience side cramps or any muscle or joint pains.
- Always warm up with stretching to avoid injury.

Some bodies are better structured for jogging then others. Yet, with any body type, there's a high risk of injury to knees, ankles, and calves because of pounding on hard surfaces.

Aerobic Dance

Degree of Difficulty: Medium–High.

Benefits:
* Full-body workout.
* Easily accessible—from health spas and community centers to home use with video and audio tapes and instructional guides.
* Entertaining, incorporating high-energy music.

Guidelines:
* Check the credentials of the instructor; he or she should have formal training or certification in physical fitness rather than just "liking to dance."
* Assess the facility: type of floor surface (wood preferred); amount of ventilation; average number in class.
* Find out about the levels of classes offered: how they differ in length of class, degree of difficulty and supervision, length of warmup and cool-down periods, frequency of supervised heart rate monitoring.
* Join the best program that offers low- to high-level classes and take responsibility for yourself. Use target heart rate to avoid overexertion; forcing yourself to "keep up" is more harmful than not dancing at all.
* Always warm up. Never just jump into a class late. If you arrive late, take time to do your own warm up first.
* Wear good, supportive shoes.

MARVELOUS MACHINES

Exercise equipment is a superior way to work out because of the intensity of the workout, but it is important that you gradually build up, so you prevent overexertion. This can be done with *interval training*.

Interval training is a fail-safe way for beginners to build their fitness levels gradually. It lets you start at your own pace and gradually increase your speed and build endurance. You use timed bouts of exercise and follow with rest periods to enable you to last the full exercise session.

Your exercise sessions start off with short bouts and gradually increase in duration, according to your progress. The exercise bouts are continued until they total 20 to 30 minutes of aerobic activity. Beginning exercisers finish with the satisfaction of knowing they completed the same workout a seasoned exerciser would, but without jeopardizing their health or motivation.

How to do Interval Training:
- Start with 3–5 minutes on a machine at a slow pace, or as your target heart rate dictates.
- Take 2–4 minutes off, but keep moving—walk around the room until your heart rate slows down.
- *Never stop completely!* This would shock your system.
- Do another 3- to 5-minute session, then stop and walk around.
- Complete 6 sessions.

As your fitness level improves, the length of each session can be increased, but continue to monitor your heart rate. Do not wait until you get symptoms of overexertion such as dizziness or nausea—these are danger signals.

Good ventilation is critical. Work out in areas with good air flow. If necessary, set up a fan. Given the oxygen demands of this high-intensity aerobic activity, make sure that you have plenty of ventilation and wear cool clothing that breathes. Evaporation of sweat is what keeps your internal body temperature regulated.

Remember: You are not in competition with anyone but yourself. There are varying levels of fitness that can be attained. Use your target heart rate as a guide to increasing the duration of your exercise session. Just the thrill of feeling and seeing yourself improve is worth every ounce of sweat.

You should strive to increase the length of your exercise

session every 2–4 weeks, but you will need to be faithful to your workout routine in order to attain this goal. This pace of advancement is not mandatory. Go at your own pace. An interval workout is the same as one long exercise session.

Equipment Incentives:
- Exercise while you watch TV.
- Get a Walkman and a set of high-energy tapes to help you keep your rhythm. Add a new tape for your collection each time you advance in your workout program.
- Combine your workout with learning by getting tapes of books, or languages you always wanted to learn. One of our patients learned Italian while she got in shape for a European vacation.
- Buy the right equipment. Too many dieters have unused stationary bikes because they didn't try them out before purchasing one.
- Try out the equipment first. Go to a well-equipped health spa on a free or low-cost trial basis and test the field, to get the feel of it with instructor supervision.
- If you have a machine that you can't relate to and it's packed away, *sell it* and start over with a new machine—one that you'll use.
- Consider how portable the machine is. For warm weather, you may want to work out outside in the fresh air.

Rowing Machine
Degree of Difficulty: Medium–High.

Benefits:
- Excellent cardiovascular training.
- Great calorie-burning exercise.
- Works upper and lower body, improving strength and mobility.

- No orthopedic injury.
- Pace and tension are easily adjusted.
- Very portable; stores in small space.
- Can be used for additional strength building exercises.

Guidelines:
- Adjust the tension of the arm pulls to the lowest level.
- Sit on the seat cushion and strap feet into stirrups. Make sure handles of the rowing arms are parallel to your foot pads.
- Position the seat up to your feet so that you're in a crouched position. Keep your back straight and grasp the handles of the rowing arms.
- Glide the set backward, straightening your legs, and pull the rowing arms until your legs are fully extended and your hands are parallel to your body. (For a full arm extension, bend your arms past your body and fully extend.)
- Return to starting position by gliding the seat forward, bending your knees and simultaneously pushing the rowing arms back to the start.
- The pace at which you row and the rowing arm tension determine the intensity of your workout. Start slow!
- Wear racquet gloves to prevent or minimize blisters.

Rebounding: Mini Trampoline for Home Use

Degree of Difficulty: Low–High.

Benefits:
- Excellent cardiovascular fitness.
- Great calorie-burning potential.
- Easily accomodates all levels of fitness.
- Develops coordination and balance.
- No injury to muscles and joints.
- Excellent alternative to walking or jogging outside.
- Easy and fun to use.
- Very portable; easy storage.

• Perfect for aerobic dance without the injury.

Guidelines:
• Set the rebounder on any flat surface, indoors or outside.
• Position yourself by a wall, as a beginner, if balance is a problem.
• Bounce moderately, creating a comfortable pace, lifting knees high.
• Follow interval training guidelines, clustering exercise bouts into one session or spreading them over 3–4 times in a day.

Stationary Bicycle

Degree of Difficulty: Low–High.

Benefits:
• Great cardiovascular training.
• Excellent calorie-burning exercise, if you pedal at sufficient speed and tension.
• Easy to use with minimal instruction.
• Easily exchanged with outdoor bicycle fun.
• Strengthens leg and back muscles.
• Readily available at most health spas.
• Very appropriate exercise for advanced pregnancy since the extra "baby weight" is not a prohibiting factor when sitting on a bike.
• Advanced technology, with computerized Lifecycles and fan bicycles (Airdyne), adds another dimension of challenge. (*Lifecycles* are computerized cycles, incorporating an interval-training workout, that enable you to individually program pace, duration, and degree of difficulty along any desired incline. *Fan Cycles,* which are relatively uncommon on the health spa scene, have long arm bars that move up and back as you pedal, giving you an upper-body workout as well. In ad-

dition, the front wheel of the bicycle has a fan generated by pedaling, to keep you cooled off as you work out.)

Guidelines:
- To properly adjust your seat height to avoid leg cramps, knee strain, and leg fatigue:

  - Sit on the seat and rotate the right pedal to the down position.
  - Place the ball of your foot on the pedal. Your leg should be fully extended. Test for a slight knee bend rather than a knee lock and adjust the height of the seat.

- If you cycle outdoors with a conventional bicycle:

  - Use a standard bicycle or adjust the gears on your ten speed to pedal with some tension.
  - Keep your speed comfortable and steady. Avoid too much gliding when the bike is working without you.
  - Invest in safety gear such as a helmet, reflectors, rear view mirror, lights, and reflective clothing for night riding.

Treadmill

Degree of Difficulty: Medium–High (depends on grade, tension, pace).

Often runners use the treadmill to gain a greater cardiovascular workout by adjusting the grade or incline of the machine to simulate running uphill. However, *walkers* can maximize their workout with a brisk stride and graduated grade and tension without risking the joint trauma caused by pounding on hard surfaces.

Benefits:
- Superb cardiovascular training.
- Excellent calorie-burning exercise.
- Great for all levels of fitness, accommodating beginners to seasoned exercisers.
- Available in motorized and manual (motorized is usually better for the beginner because there's less tension and the speed and grade are easy to adjust; manual machines are more appealing to the advanced treadmiller because of the greater challenge of motorizing it yourself).
- Reduces body injury.
- Available at many health spas, especially those emphasizing cardiovascular fitness.

How to Use:
- Adjust the tension (especially if you are a beginner) to the lowest level.
- Begin walking at a comfortable pace; you should not be breathless. Use your target heart rate as a guide to speed up or slow down.
- If your treadmill is motorized, adjust the grade to a slight incline or no incline as a beginner, and gradually increase the grade as your fitness level improves, and set the pace at a comfortable yet brisk level.

Nordic Track: Simulated Cross-Country Skiing

Degree of Difficulty: High.

Benefits:
- Best cardiovascular training.
- Best calorie-burning exercise.
- No orthopedic injury; no shock to joints and muscles.
- Works upper and lower body (especially buttocks); can adjust tension for greater strength building and higher intensity.
- Builds coordination and rhythm.

Guidelines:
- Slip feet into stirrups on skiis, which glide along track.
- Lean slightly forward, balancing pelvis against pelvic cushion.
- Grasp handles on arm pulley.
- Position arms and legs in opposite positions (i.e., left leg forward, right leg back—toe bends up—right arm pulled up, left arm pulled back).
- Then switch positions, gliding opposite leg forward and simultaneously pulling arm pulley, switching arm positions.
- If you struggle with either leg or arm movement, decrease tension on either or both gauges.
- The goal is to develop a comfortable, gliding stride. The opposition of arm and leg movement keeps your balance while you lean forward against the pelvic cushion.
- Handle bars are also attached so you can start out just learning leg coordination, yet in the long run, it's easier to balance when the machine is used as designed with arms and legs in opposition. It's a natural stride, like walking. Don't outthink your stride, just glide!

SKILL SPORT AEROBICS

Skill sports include tennis, racquetball, squash, handball, skiing, basketball, volleyball, and so forth.

Degree of Difficulty: Low–High.

Benefits:
- Easily combined wth a more regular aerobic routine.
- Add variety and excitement, challenging a partner or joining forces with a team.
- Considered play rather than workout.

Guidelines:
- Play as frequently as possible to improve skill, since skill level determines aerobic intensity. (Go to p. 68.)

Calorie Burn with Various Aerobic Activities

Calories Burned in 30 Minutes of Activity

Activity	Calorie/ min/lb	120-lb Person	150-lb Person
Aerobic dance	.038	137	171
Basketball	.068	245	306
Bedmaking	.026	94	117
Bicycling	.071	256	320
Canoeing (2.5 mi/hr)	.019	68	86
Chopping wood	.048	173	216
Cleaning windows	.028	101	126
Cross-country skiing	.078	281	351
Gardening (weeding)	.039	140	176
Golf	.030	108	135
Handball	.076	274	342
Horseback riding (trot)	.049	176	220
Ironing	.037	133	166
Jogging (5 mi/hr)	.057	205	256
Laundry (hanging clothes)	.047	169	212
Washing floors	.030	108	135
Painting house	.055	198	248
Rowing (4 mi/hr)	.072	259	324
Running (7 mph)	.094	338	423
Sawing wood	.048	173	216
Shoveling snow	.053	191	238
Skiing (alpine)	.064	230	288
Squash	.060	216	270
Swimming (crawl)	.032	115	144
Table tennis	.034	122	153
Tennis	.045	162	202
Walking	.049	176	220

To find the number of calories that you burn during activity: (1) multiply the number in the first column by your weight, then (2) multiply that number by the number of minutes you perform the activity.

Data derived from "The LEARN Program for Weight Control," K. Brownell, Ph.D., copyright 1985.

- Couple these games with other aerobic activities to equal half an hour at least 3 times per week.
- Try to stay in continuous motion and minimize non-active time.

WHY YOU NEED TO EXERCISE FROM DAY 1 OF YOUR DIET

To fine-tune your metabolism: Calorie restriction can reduce your calorie-burning power by causing your metabolic rate to drop as much as 10–15 percent. You can burn fewer calories, even though you cut them to burn more. This could cause you to stop losing weight or to lose very slowly. Exercise raises your metabolic rate by 10–15 percent to offset this loss of burning power.

To preserve your muscle: Fat is the only loss you can afford on a diet. Muscle losses undermine your metabolism and reduce your burning power. Exercise preserves muscle during a diet, to insure that you burn only fat.

To balance your fat-to-muscle ratio: At the end of your diet, your fat-to-muscle status is of primary concern. It will determine how many calories you can eat at maintenance without gaining weight. Studies showed that two people of the same height, weight, and sex can eat the same number of calories at the end of a diet, and one will gain while the other will not. Why? The one who won't gain has a low-fat–high-muscle body.

To gain oxygen for fat burn: When you exercise, you use more oxygen. For fat to be burned, oxygen is necessary. With aerobic exercise, you can expect greater burn of stored fat.

To increase intestinal motility: Food passes through your intestines better when exercise is a regular routine. An average nonexerciser can take 24 hours to complete one digestive cycle, an obese nonexerciser can take up to 48 hours. Too slow! Food that lingers in your intestines can stagnate and lead to digestive disorders or increase your risk of bowel cancer. Exercise speeds food transit time through your intestines. Athletes show intestinal motility of 4 to 6 hours to complete digestion.

To regulate your appetite: Loss of appetite follows a good workout. When activity levels are low, studies show that people increase their calorie intake.

To fight anxiety and depression: Endorphins are opiatelike chemicals produced in your brain that modulate pain and moods. Exercise increases their production, leaving you with a euphoric feeling. Your circulation is improved and this creates a sense of well-being. Therapists are beginning to prescribe aerobic exercise and dance as therapy against anxiety and depression, with one study boasting an 82 percent success rate in hard-to-treat patients.

To reduce stress: Fifty to 75 percent of all organic illnesses are aggravated by or related to stress. Stress stimulates your sympathetic nervous system, speeding your heart rate, increasing your blood pressure, and contributing to cardiovascular disease. Exercise reverses the stress response by reducing your heart rate, lowering your blood pressure, and improving your sense of control.

To lose fat for disease prevention: High body fat has been linked to most of our major lifestyle diseases, including hypertension, heart disease, diabetes, and cancer—specifically colon cancer in men and breast cancer in women. Since exercise reduces body fat, you reduce the risk of acquiring these diseases by exercising. Recent studies show that exercise can significantly reduce the risk of heart attack by improving heart and lung function and increasing the concentration of HDL, a protein that removes cholesterol from your blood and is associated with a lower risk of coronary heart disease.

To increase your energy output: Movement requires energy. The more you move, the more energy you use, which means more calories burned.

In addition to its metabolic benefits, exercise is the best *behavior substitute* for eating. Go for thermic action from the first day of your diet. Don't cut calories without adding exercise.

CARDIOVASCULAR CONDITIONING

Aerobic exercise improves the power of your heart and circulation. When the activity is performed regularly and for sufficient periods of time, it can produce beneficial physiological changes. Your body becomes a better machine. It can take in, transport, and use oxygen at an increased rate. Your heart becomes a better pump, pushing more blood out with each stroke, and it rests longer between beats. Distribution and blood flow in your lungs and working muscles are enhanced, and slowing of your heart rate (pulse) occurs both at rest and at any given level of activity. As a result, your cardiovascular system operates more efficiently.

To achieve cardiovascular conditioning, certain conditions must be met:

- *Duration:* The exercise must be performed at a suitable level of intensity for 20–30 minutes (not counting warmups or cool-downs).
- *Frequency:* The exercise should be performed at least 3 times per week, preferably on alternate days.
- *Intensity:* The exercise must be strenuous enough for you to reach a level of exertion that is about 70–85 percent of your maximum heart rate.

The most suitable sports for cardiovascular conditioning are the ones that require repeated and continuous movement—running, swimming, cycling, brisk walking, rowing, rope skipping, running in place, stationary cycling, basketball, handball, racquetball, squash, skating, hockey, cross-county skiing, soccer, and hiking.

Other sports might not be adequate for cardiovascular

conditioning if they allow long pauses between action or the movement takes place in brief spurts. In the same way that you want to keep the heat constant in your eating style, you need to keep the heat steady with your exercise. Low-heat exercises include baseball, softball, golf, and bowling.

Calisthenics that emphasize slow bending, stretching, and graceful movement will not provide cardiovascular benefits as well as continuous, rhythmic calisthenics that are performed at a higher level of intensity.

TAKING YOUR TARGET HEART RATE

When you exercise, your heart beats harder, keeping a good supply of oxygen-carrying blood circulating to all of the muscles in your body. Exercising properly means regulating how hard your heart beats without overexerting it. This can be achieved by measuring your heart rate (pulse), then adjusting how vigorously you exercise (intensity) and the length of time you exercise (duration).

A formula used to determine your *maximal heart rate* is:

220 − your age = maximal heart rate (MHR)

This is the maximum degree of heart *overexertion* and is dangerous to sustain during exercise.

The best level for exercise is known as your *target heart rate zone*, which is 70–85 pecent of your maximal heart rate.

The formula used to find your target heart rate (THR) is:

Maximal Heart Rate × 0.7 = 70% intensity
Maximal Heart Rate × 0.85 = 85% intensity

As you condition your heart and body with regular aerobic exercise, your heart rate will decrease, meaning that your heart is stronger and pumping more efficiently. This also means you can work out more vigorously and for a longer stretch of time and still stay within your target heart rate. This is an indication of cardiovascular fitness. As a beginner, work in the lower range of the target heart rate zone until your cardiovascular system becomes stronger and your body becomes better conditioned.

How to Take Your Heart Rate:
- Find the pulse in the side of your neck, under your jawbone, with your index and middle fingers.
- Count the number of beats for 6 seconds.
- Add a zero to the end of that number and you will have your heartbeats per minute.

When to Take Your Heart Rate:
- If you are just beginning an aerobic exercise program, you need to pace yourself, checking your heart rate frequently.
- Using interval training, check your heart rate immediately following each exercise session. Your heart rate will begin to drop soon after you stop working. If your heart rate is not up to your target heart rate zone, increase your speed or intensity of exercise. If your

Calculated Target Heart Rates by Age

Age in Years	Maximal Heart Rate	Target Heart Rate Zone 70–85% Intensity	Beats per 10 seconds
20	200	140–170	23–28
25	195	136–166	23–28
30	190	133–162	22–27
35	185	130–157	22–26
40	180	126–153	21–26
45	175	122–149	20–25
50	170	119–144	20–24
55	165	116–140	19–23
60	160	112–136	19–23
65	155	108–132	18–22

heart rate is greater than your target heart rate zone, slow your pace but *do not stop.*
- As you increase the length of your exercise session, check your heart rate periodically to insure that you're not overexerting your heart.

WARM-UPS

Use these warm-ups *before* any aerobic exercise.
Warm-ups are a preconditioning *must!*

Purpose:
- Gets blood circulating better.
- Warms your muscles and joints.
- Gently stretches your muscles to prevent injury.
- Slightly elevates heart rate.
- Prepares your body for a workout.

1. Spine Stretch (back, hip, shoulder).
   Kneel on the floor, then sit down on your heels and with a flat back, stretch your arms overhead and lean forward with your face toward the floor and arms stretching in front. Hold for count of 25.
2. Hang Loose (spine, hamstrings).
   Stand with legs spread slightly wider than the width of shoulders, knees slightly bent. Gradually curl torso, letting arms hang by your feet. Hold for count of 10. Roll back up and repeat 3 times. With each repetition, your arms will hang lower to the floor.
3. Side Stretch (waist, shoulders).
   Stand with legs spread shoulder width apart, knees slightly bent, toes straight ahead. Stretch arms overhead, clasp thumbs together, and gently lean to your right side and hold for 6 counts. Return to center. Lean to the left side and hold for 6 counts. Repeat 3 times.

4. Side Lunge (hamstrings, groin).

Stand with legs spread slightly wider than shoulder width. Point right foot slightly out. Extend arms to each side at shoulder height. Keeping hips facing forward, gently lean to your right; make sure that your right knee is extending directly over your toe. Hold for 6 counts. Return to center. Repeat to left side. Repeat 3 times.

5. Head Rolls (neck, spine).

Stand straight, knees slightly bent. Allow your shoulders to drop slightly (being careful not to round shoulders and back). Gently drop your head forward, chin into your chest. Slowly roll your head around to your right, then to the back, then to the left, completing a full circle. Reverse direction of rotation and repeat. Repeat 3 times.

6. Arm-Wrist Stretch (arms, shoulder, wrists).

Stand erect, arms outstretched to both sides. Make 20 small circles in the air with your arms, rotating forward. Repeat, reversing circle motion.

Arms outstretched, bend wrists downward (hold 4 counts), then flex upward—pointing fingers up (hold 4 counts). Repeat 10 times.

7. Frog Stretch (hips, groin).

Sit on the floor, back erect. Pull your legs in with the soles of your feet touching. Gently press your knees toward the floor with your elbows. *Do not* bounce or force. Hold for count of 6. Repeat 3 times.

8. Spread Stretch (hamstring, back, side).

Sit on the floor. Extend and spread your legs, keeping your back straight. Lean forward with flat back and extend arms in front of you. Gradually walk your fingers along the floor, reaching farther. Hold for 10 counts. Relax and repeat 3 times.

Return to center, back erect. Place left hand on inside thigh of your right leg. Stretch your right arm overhead and, facing forward, lean to your left. Reach for your left toe. You will feel a nice side stretch.

Keep your torso elongated; do not crouch. Hold for
6 counts. Return to center. Repeat to right side, placing your right hand on your left thigh and reach
toward your right leg with your left arm. Repeat 3
times.

9. Lower Leg Stretch (calf, ankles).

Lean at arms length against a wall. Place your
right leg forward, toes straight ahead, knee bent.
Extend your left leg back, heel flat on the floor, toe
forward. Lean toward the wall, bending elbows and
supporting body with your forward leg. You will feel
an elongated stretch of your calf and ankle. Hold for
8 counts. Reverse legs and repeat. Repeat 3 times.

10. Ankle Rotation.

Supporting yourself against a wall, extend right
leg slightly off the ground in front of you. Gently
rotate your ankle in 5 small circles. Reverse direction and repeat. Change legs and repeat ankle rotation with your left leg.

COOL-DOWNS

Use these cool-downs *after* any aerobic workout. They prevent lactic acid buildup in your muscles, which causes sore-
ness. Cool-downs cause lactic acid breakdown into carbon
dioxide and water as soon as oxygen reaches your muscles
in the cooldown phase. This avoids those groans from pain
the morning after exercise.

1. Immediately following your aerobic workout, walk
   around the room for 2–4 minutes until your heart
   rate gradually returns to normal.
2. Lower Leg Stretch
   Lean at arms length against a wall. Place your right
   leg forward, toes straight ahead, knee bent. Extend
   your left leg back, heel flat on the floor, toes forward.
   Lean toward the wall, bending your elbows and sup-

porting your body with your forward leg. You will feel an elongated stretch of your calf and ankle. Hold for 10 counts. Reverse legs and repeat. Repeat 3 times.

3. Full Body Stretch

   Lie flat on your back, tucking in your stomach and your pelvis toward the floor so as to eliminate the space between your back and the floor. Extend your arms overhead. Stretch your arms and legs simultaneously, pulling as far as they'll go. Feel yourself elongate. Hold for 10 counts. Relax. Repeat 3 times.

4. Fetal Tuck

   Turn on your right side and curl up your body, pulling your legs toward your chest, head down, and holding your knees with your arms. Hold for 10 counts. Turn to your left side and repeat.

5. Leg Extension

   Lie flat on your back and bend your left leg, foot flat on the floor. Slowly bend your right knee into your chest, hold for 6 counts, then extend your leg straight up, perpendicular to the floor. Support your leg by holding on to your ankle. Gently pull the leg forward. *Do not force.* Hold for 10 counts. Reverse legs and repeat.

6. Total Body Relaxation.

   Lie flat on your back, placing a chair or stool under your leg. Rest your lower legs on the chair (bending at the knees). Rest your arms at your sides. Close your eyes. Concentrate on your breathing. Relax for 2–4 minutes.

SELECTING THE RIGHT SHOES

Ordinary shoes do not provide enough support for the stress from the impact of steady walking. As the saying goes, "If the shoe fits, wear it," and when the shoe is for walking, be sure it fits well.

The two most important aspects of fit are *comfort* and

support. Shoes serve as a buffer between the bones and muscles of your body and the uncharitable ground, regardless of the surface.

Look for a shoe with a thick, rounded, slightly elevated heel to cushion against the shock and stress of impact. The heel back and ankle rim should be reinforced for ankle support and to prevent your foot from pushing out the back of the shoe after repeated heel strikes.

Be sure there is a space the width of your thumb between your big toe and the front of the shoe, and be careful that your big toe does not touch the top of the shoe. Look for a toe box that is reinforced with strong material to keep your toes from stretching and pushing out at the front.

Try bending the sole of the shoe—it should be flexible. The soles should also have adequate cushioning for absorbing shock. The shoes should have soft, built-in arch support. The larger person should buy a shoe that is somewhat firmer and offers good heel and forefront support.

Check to see that the lacing strip is long enough to allow for tension adjustments and good fit control around the entire foot. Nylon material is better than leather, since nylon breathes more freely and prevents excessive sweating, which can create blisters. Improperly sewn seams can also cause blisters, so select a pair of shoes that are sewn symmetrically.

No matter what type of walking shoes you buy, wear them with cotton socks, and wear the socks while trying on your shoes, to insure the best fit. Never buy a pair of shoes with the idea of breaking them in. Take a walk around the store or jog in place to test the fit. Make sure the shoe isn't rubbing uncomfortably against any part of your foot.

HOW FAT ARE YOUR FAVORITE ATHLETES?

Body fat studies of athletes show a high degree of difference in percent of body fat in different sports. Overall, females are higher-fat than their male counterparts. Also, performance in a sport in which your body is moving through space, as in running and gymnastics, improves with a lower percent of body fat. On the other hand, athletes in sports in which performance is enhanced by the force of body weight, such as discus throwers, shot putters, or football linemen, improve with a slightly higher percent of body fat. Find your favorite sport in the following table, to find out what it takes in muscle. Notice, too, that older athletes in the same sport often have lower percentages of body fat, which means you don't have to settle for a fatter body as you age.

Sport	Age	Wt	Percent of Body Fat	
			Male	Female
Baseball	21	183	14%	
	21	183	12	
	27	194	13	
Basketball	19	138		21%
	19	141		27
Center	28	240	7	
Forward	25	213	9	
Guard	25	184	11	
Football				
Defensive Back	17–23	170	12	
Offensive Back	17–23	176	12	
Linebacker	17–23	192	13	
Offensive Lineman	17–23	218	19	
Defensive Lineman	17–23	215	19	
Quarterbacks and Kickers	24	198	14	
Gymnasts	20	152	5	
	19	127		24
	20	113		16
Ice Hockey	23	170	13	
	26	191	15	
Jockeys	31	111	14	

Sport	Age	Wt	Percent of Body Fat	
			Male	Female
Racquetball	25	177	8	
	23	150		14
Skiing	26	165	7	
Alpine	21	154	14	
	20	129		21
Cross-Country	21	146	13	
	26	152	10	
	20	123		16
	24	130		22
Soccer	26	166	10	
Speed Skating	21	168	11	
Swimming	21	174	5	
	22	174	9	
	19	140		26
	19	147		24
Tennis	42	170	16	
	39	122		20
Track and Field	21	158	4	
Runners	23	142	6	
	26	146	8	
	40–49	158	11	
	50–59	148	11	
	60–69	148	11	
	70–75	147	14	
	20	116		19
	32	126		15
Discus	26	243	16	
	21	156		25
Jumpers and Hurdlers	20	130		20
Shot Put	22	278	20	
	22	172		28
Volleyball	19	132		25
	20	144		21

Sport	Age	Wt	Percent of Body Fat	
			Male	Female
Weight Lifting	25	170	10	
	26	202	16	
	28	194	8	
Wrestling	23	174	14	
	26	180	9	
	27	166	11	

Adapted from J. H. Wilmore et al. *Ann. NY Academy Science* 301:764–776, 1977.

NINE

BEHAVIOR MODIFICATION

The purpose of behavior modification is to change the habits that have been harming you into habits that will enhance your life.

Habits are learned behaviors, and as such, can be unlearned. A chain of habits string together to make up that unique territory known as your "style" or lifestyle.

Your lifestyle includes everything you do from the time you wake in the morning until you turn in at night. It's what you eat, how fast you eat, how much you eat, and why. It's how you exercise—if you exercise. It's all the choices you make and why you make them. Lifestyle is self-imposed stress. It's management and mismanagement of time. It's how hard you work and play, how seriously you take your health, and how well you sleep. Your lifestyle is the sum total of all the aspects of your life.

Habits are the keys to success, because they can take on an automatic life of their own. They've had daily rehearsals over the years, and cling with the tenacity of epoxy, even if they are bad habits.

Unlearning bad habits and replacing them with good ones is a challenging course. It's a process that removes old obstacles and releases new energy to help you cope. The positive results flow over into all the other areas of your life.

IDEAL BODY *WHAT?*

From now on, think of Ideal Body Weight as Ideal Body Fat.

Not all weight is fat. Water and muscle weigh on the scale. As a result, Ideal Body Weight tables are not accurate indicators of your body composition. They do not show the amount of water, muscle, or fat in your body. They lump water, muscle, and fat together and assume they're in the right proportions for a given height. That's like allowing you to confuse the ingredients in a recipe for sauce. Let's say the sauce calls for 1 cup of water, 1 cup of tomatoes, and 1 *teaspoon* of salt. Instead, you use 1 teaspoon of water, 1 cup of tomatoes, and 1 *cup* of salt. You wouldn't serve the sauce to a friend, and we can't serve Ideal Body Weight to you.

BEATING THE BODY WEIGHT TRAP

If you have been seeking a goal called Ideal Body Weight, you have been falling into a trap. You can reach Ideal Body Weight in a number of different ways, but if you haven't lost fat, you've wasted your time, money, and emotional energy supporting weight loss that won't last.

At Ideal Body Weight, if you haven't come close to your Ideal Body Fat, your metabolism will still be sluggish and fat-preserving. If you haven't increased your lean muscle mass and burning power, when you try to maintain your weight, you'll find you can't do it.

When you lose fat and gain muscle, you can weigh more than the Ideal Body Weight tables say is right for your frame. You can be slim and weigh more than a fatter person, because muscle is heavier than fat. In other words, you can reach Ideal body Fat weighing more than you had set as your goal because you increased your lean muscle mass. But with a lower percent of body fat, you'll be leaner and fit smaller sizes.

LOOSENING UP IN YOUR CLOTHES

A realistic diet goal is to forget about the numbers game and *loosen up* in your clothing.

For men whose fat deposits occur mostly in the upper body, a shirt is a good gauge for successful fat loss.

For women whose fat deposits occur mostly in the lower body as waist and hip girth, a pair of slacks is a good gauge for successful fat loss.

Remember: You can't rush fat loss. Fat is lost proportionately from every area of your body, even though it seems it only deposits in spots.

Chart your progress by looser clothing, and gaining a leaner, firmer overall body appearance. Plan realistic *fat loss* of 1 percent of your body weight per week. Remember: You are losing fat, not weight. You will find, to your surprise, that fat loss "looks like" more weight loss than the scale will register. Fat loss leads to a leaner body image.

Often you will notice that at the end of a diet, people look haggard and baggy. This does not happen with fat loss; it happens with muscle wasting and water losses. Therefore, every pound of fat you lose is going to make you look better.

TRACKING YOUR PROGRESS

Weight _____ pounds
Neck circumference _____ inches
Upper arm circumference _____ inches
Hips _____ inches
Waist _____ inches
Thighs _____ inches
Calf _____ inches
Ankles _____ inches

Use the measurements above to chart your fat loss progress. Every two weeks, measure yourself and rechart your percent of body fat (see Chapter 2). Your rate of change will be gradual at first, because you are losing fat. Change will occur! You must continue even if you show only slight measurement changes.

YOUR SCALE

Don't rate your weight loss.

Your scale is your worst enemy on a diet. If you must weigh yourself, here's how to do it: *Put your scale in a box and stand on top of it. Look down.* (Congratulate yourself on your progress and go back to your diet and exercise.)

Your scale tells you nothing about your percent of body fat or percent of muscle mass.

It will tell you about water displacement, which is common on a diet.

Your scale sets you up for failure! Here's how it works:

Setup number 1—false sense of success: You had a good day. You followed your diet, did your exercise and were active. You step on the scale and what's this? *You lost 3 pounds.* Some of the losses are water displacement that will come right back. If you don't know this, you might think you're doing great, and you might go for a dessert tomorrow. Or you might think you don't need as much exercise so you'll slack off. *You would subvert your whole diet.*

Setup number 2—false sense of failure: It was warm out and you were active. You adhered to your diet and did your workout. You even played tennis with a friend. You drank a lot of water when you came home. You step on the scale and horrors! *You gained 3 pounds.* But the gain is water and will balance back out. If you don't know this, you might think your diet is flopping and stop out of frustration. *You would subvert your whole diet.*

Setup number 3—false fear of failure: You seem to be losing fat regularly because you are thinner around the middle and your clothes are looser and you feel lighter. You step on the scale and you've barely lost a pound in two weeks. But your present weight includes a gain in muscle mass that will improve your burning power. If you don't know this, you might think there's something wrong with you. Back to negative thinking. Are you sick? Should you go for a checkup? Can you trust this diet? Is your body thermostat off? Is your scale broken or what? How can you be thinner without showing it? Do you have a secret illness? Typical, isn't it, just when you were making progress. *Forget it*. You'll get so stressed, *you'll subvert your whole diet.*

If you must weigh yourself, do it once a week. Put your scale in a box and take it out every Monday morning. Only on a weekly basis will the numbers play your way.

Don't rely on your scale. Rely on your better body feelings.

WATER: KEEPING YOUR FAT REMOVAL MOVING

If you give up your addiction to the scale and replace that impulse with drinking water, you'll be breaking two of the worst habits of bad dieting.

Most dieters don't drink enough water. They don't think about water. Or they think they retain water, so losing some will be all right. Wrong.

Half your body weight is water. Eighty percent of the liquid substance of 75 trillion body cells is water. Replacing the water daily, keeping it circulating through your system, is the best thing you can do for your health.

It regulates your body temperature.

It washes out toxic wastes.

It maintains the proper volume and pressure of your blood.

It supplies oxygen and nutrients to your muscles and organs.

It facilitates chemical reactions.

It lubricates your joints.

It protects your tissues.

Water is more important than food.

You could survive for weeks without a morsel of food, but you wouldn't last longer than one or two days without water.

If you were stranded on a desert island and could have your choice of food, your favorite movie star, or a gallon of water, and you were left alone a day or two to think it over, you'd choose water.

Your body water is unevenly distributed. Solid structures like your skeleton contain little water, while your organs, muscles, and other metabolically active tissue have a much higher water content. Muscles are "wetter," being 72 percent water, whereas fat is only 20 percent water. Men have slightly more water than women, with 50 to 60 percent of their body mass as water, compared to 50 percent for women. And we all grow drier as we age and need more water.

Some dieters suffer from water retention and think if they reduce their water intake, their bodies will have less water to hold in. They may even resort to diuretics, failing to realize that water itself is the best diuretic on the market! Having plenty of water in your system discourages your body from sending out panic signals to save water.

Your water intake must equal your water loss.

You lose approximately half a gallon of water per day. When you exercise, the temperature rises outside, or you have a fever, your water losses can dramatically increase.

On an average day, you lose:

- 2 cups of water through sweating.
- 1 quart and 1 cup of water through body excretions.
- 1 cup of water through breathing.

Everyone knows we are supposed to drink between 8 to 10 glasses of water per day, but not many people do. Part of the problem is remembering to drink. Most dieters only drink when they are thirsty, but by then 1- to 2-percent dehydration has occured. You can't afford to wait to be thirsty before you reach for your water glass.

When you diet, you must drink at least 2 quarts of water per day.

Water is as essential as exercise while you are dieting. It fills you up, keeps hunger at bay, acts as a diuretic, and protects you from dehydration.

Don't let a day of your diet go by without 8 glasses of water.

Since water is the major component of most of your favorite drinks, you can meet your water needs by drinking any of the following beverages: springwater, seltzer water, club soda, diet soda, juice, juice spritzers, coffee, and tea. (Caffeinated beverages cause you to lose fluid, so limit the amount of coffee and tea that you drink.)

GAINING MENTAL MUSCLE

You cannot overlook the importance of the emotional energy you invest in a diet program. Psychologists cite common problems among dieters who have tried diets that failed and consequently fear another failure. Being very overweight is not necessarily caused by psychological problems, but such problems can emerge as people carry too much weight too long. This negative emotional input includes loss of self-esteem, poor body image, resticted socializing, limited mobility, and lack of assertiveness, especially in the overweight female who develops obesity.

Your "body image" is formed in large part by what others think about the way you look and how they treat you as a result. Descriptive terms like "tall" or "beautiful" are essentially culture-bound and subjective. In a tribe of short natives, a 6-foot-tall man would be considered a giant. In a tribe of bald natives, a woman with long curly hair would not be considered beautiful or acceptable. And yet "fat" seems to carry the most weight when it comes to feeling like an outsider in our society. The media barrage us with thinner images every year, to such extremes of fatlessness for women that half our teenage girls are on diets by the time they are twelve or thirteen. The message that comes through the media is "Thin is beautiful, fat is ugly. Thin is socially acceptable, fat is not." This message—realistic or not—slowly becomes ingrained and curbs our emotional freedom. Fat becomes frightening, a case for avoidance.

Fat Eyes: Overweight people often begin thinking of how they look only from the neck up. Taking a body inventory becomes a painful process. Body language becomes protective. Body trust is not great. Attention to the body is a source of unhappiness. Looking into the mirror means looking at fat, so full-length mirrors are avoided. Sometimes fat eyes become so critical they remain even after a successful diet when a thinner image is maintained. In our exercise clinics, we found many women going to great lengths to avoid mirrors, choosing to exercise in corners where they couldn't see themselves.

Fat Colors: Body hiding becomes second nature. Dark colors are preferred over light tones. Dull shades take the place of bright ones. A wardrobe of fat clothes shows loose-fitting dresses or baggy shirts, oversized sweat suits and caftans. Shirts are worn loose and long, instead of tucked in. Belts are avoided. It's very common for dieters to support an attitude of failure by keeping a wardrobe of fat clothes around, just in case . . .

Fat Talk: Body talk centers on self-criticism. "I'm not. I can't. I don't. I won't try. It's not worth it." Self-trust is low. The inner voice is always saying something negative.

Starting a diet program with negative beliefs about yourself is setting yourself up for failure. In the case of your emotions and self-image, it's vital to remember that your brain remembers what you told it yesterday and runs on that today. If you've spent years berating yourself, that's what your brain knows and projects forward.

Today, you can start giving yourself a more positive attitude. Begin thinking of yourself as successful and appreciated today. Tell yourself you're great. Even if you don't believe it, do it anyway. It works by itself. Your brain only knows what you tell it, and it will remember tomorrow what you tell it today.

Every time you express a negative thought to yourself, cancel it and rephrase it. Change it to something positive. If your inner voice is disagreeing, that's only your brain burning off its old stuff. Ignore it. Say something positive. Start today to rewrite your emotional history.

Simultaneously, stop warring with your body. It's the only one you've got, so treat it like royalty. Body hatred never accomplishes anything positive. And remember: Your body is very forgiving. Regardless of the things you've done in the past with bad dieting or poor nutrition, when you take positve steps, your body responds positively. We've seen many examples like the following:

> Mr. N was an airline pilot who joined the program because he feared being grounded. For Mr. N, not passing a flight physical meant not having a job. Concerned about his high blood pressure as well as his weight, he was determined to change his lifestyle. Twenty-six pounds lighter, Mr. N passed his flight physical with flying colors. With decreased weight, his high blood pressure was controlled. Now an obvious example of health and fitness, Mr. N says, "If I knew good health could feel so great, I would have done this years ago."

You don't have to deprive yourself of fitness because you haven't experienced it before. Instead of going for rapid, unhealthy, and fleeting weight loss, go for better body balance inside, where it counts, in your fat-to-muscle ratio. The rest follows naturally.

CREATING YOUR DIET ENVIRONMENT

The minute anyone mentions a diet, the first thought that follows is deprivation, especially if the diet is low in fat. But your thermic program will not deprive you; it's full of variety and will satisfy your hunger and cravings. Even so, that doesn't change how you've perceived diets in the past.

Therefore, for the first part of your diet, you might think you're being deprived. It's important to change that way of thinking.

Replace the sense of palate deprivation—real or imagined—with sensory stimulus.

Introduce color, music, laughter, scents, and sensory pleasures into your diet environment.

- *Feel* confident that you are going to reach maintenance in the best shape yet. You have the power on your side. All you have to do is use it.
- *Hear* yourself sounding more confident and self-supportive every day. Give yourself constant, positive reinforcement.
- *Taste* the freshness in your food as you eat. Chew slowly and let the sensations linger. In the same way that fat blunts your appreciation of lighter foods, it dulls the sense of taste. With a low-fat diet, you'll find your taste buds awakening.
- *Smell* the fresh food aromas as you cook low-fat. Fat tends to blunt your perception of lighter scents, but going low-fat will revive your more subtle senses.
- *See* yourself becoming more fit with exercise. You will be growing leaner and stronger, and you will feel more energized, more alive, and more in control of the other aspects of your diet as you adapt to a regular exercise routine. Watch for it.
- *Believe* in your ability to succeed. Make positive changes today, to affect tomorrow positively.

Charging Up Your Kitchen

The best-laid plans for your diet can go astray in your kitchen. Kitchens have their own history in our awareness of growing up and coming to terms with the trials of the world. Kitchens were places where mothers soothed us into comfort and security with the smells of food cooking and cakes baking. Kitchens were our resource for something satisfying to eat when we were kids with bruised knees or bruised egos.

A famous writer once said that when he was looking for a good story he didn't go into the den where the men were serving brandy and cigars, he went into the kitchen where gossip was being traded over cakes and coffee.

Your kitchen should not look like a bomb shelter during your diet. If you strip your kitchen to a bare minimum you'll probably find yourself wandering in a daze to someone else's kitchen for a break. A deprived kitchen is a statement that you are depriving yourself. Don't set yourself up for deprivation. Just because you are stripping the fat from your foods, you don't have to strip the life from your kitchen to do it.

- Replace your fat-full foods with a bonanza of colorful carbohydrates.
- Use colored bowls to store your healthy diet foods.
- Keep flowers in the kitchen, or sweet-smelling herbs.
- Set up a spice rack next to the stove.
- Place colored mats under your water glass.
- Put up mouth-watering pictures of fat-free foods.
- If you have a family that won't go fat-free with you, paste white paper over their seductive boxes of fat foods and snacks, so their foods look generic, not yours.
- Fresh smells and color will wake up your senses, and substitute for the false feelings of deprivation you associate with dieting.

Boosting Your Mood

- Treat yourself to a crystal karafe and serve your water from it at the table.
- Keep a basket of potpourri on your coffee table and by your bed.
- Use music to soothe you in every room.
- Put scented soaps in the bathroom. Bathe in candlelight and sip lemon water.

- Powder your bed sheets and pillows with a fresh scent.
- Place something red in every room. A flower, a pillow, a red phone, a red hat. When you look at it, think: "I'm doing something aggressive to improve my life."
- Tape a party and play it back at home, listening without eating.
- Use scented candles in every room.
- Keep your sneakers by the door. Think of them as art, like Van Gogh's old shoes. Use them every day.
- Lemonize your sink.
- Advertise yourself with a sign that says: "I'm not on a diet, I'm on a life-improvement program."

Set up your environment the night before you start dieting. When you wake to the first day of your program, you'll feel a surge of pleasure. Keep your environment highly charged to avoid thoughts that you are punishing yourself with a diet. You are treating yourself to a better life.

EATING LOW-FAT

Eating low-fat doesn't have to be bland or boring if you use your ingenuity to improve the flavor of your meals.

- Experiment with herbs and spices in fresh or dried varieties. Some of our favorites are rosemary on chicken, dill on fish, cinnamon on carrots, nutmeg on cottage cheese, and curry on fruit.
- Use lemon juice and vinegar to add moistness and flavor when you sauté.
- Use a dash of mustard to mix with tuna or salmon, as a substitute for mayonnaise, baste on chicken or fish, mix into salads with vinegar for a hot vinaigrette.
- Use yogurt—with vegetables and spices—as a substitute for sour cream. (See Emergency Thermic Boosters for a creamy yogurt spread.) Use yogurt on your baked potato, or as a mix for macaroni salads. For a great

salad dressing try combining yogurt with a package of dry dressing like Hidden Valley Ranch, Good Seasons, or Knoors Soup Mix, a combination that can also be used as a dip.

- Buttermilk can be substituted for yogurt for a smooth salad dressing at 5 calories per teaspoon.
- Use tomato or vegetable juice for cooking meat and steaming or stewing vegetables.
- Poach fish in diluted dry wine—the heat will evaporate the alcohol and leave the flavor.
- Use broth or bouillon to moisten meats and fish, to sauté vegetables, to stir-fry and as a base for low-fat vegetable soups.
- Put low-fat cottage cheese in a blender to make a low-calorie dip or spread. To spice it up, add dehydrated soup mix or finely chopped fresh herbs and vegetables such as chives, parsley, red peppers, and cucumber.
- Mix low-fat cottage cheese in a blender with tuna or salmon to add moistness.
- Make your own refreshing water-based drinks with seltzer water for sparkle and lemon, lime, grapefruit, cranberry, or orange for a fruit boost.
- Use canned tomatoes as the base for low-fat tomato sauces.
- Boil rice in broth or bouillon for added flavor.
- Add sugar-free gelatins like strawberry or raspberry to applesauce for absolutely fabulous spreads!

WHY YOU EAT WHAT YOU EAT

Protein

The word protein comes from a Greek word that means "of first importance." It is a constituent of every cell, and the functional element in glandular secretions, enzymes, and hormones. Protein is essential for tissue growth and repair, regulation of your fluid balance, and stimulation of anti-body formation to combat infections.

It is particularly critical for dieters who are cutting back on calories to consider the quality and quantity of protein they need to meet daily requirements.

Proteins are complex substances made up of a series of amino acids or structural building blocks that are chemically bound together. There are 20 or more different amino acids that occur naturally, with the amino acid combinations creating the nature of different proteins. This is the same as forming different words from different combinations of letters. If you were in the middle of the ocean in a sinking boat with a plane flying overhead, and you had only six flag letters to signal the plane, you might spell R-E-S-C-U-E or S-E-C-U-R-E. The arrangement of the letters is of first importance. It's the same with amino acid combinations that form proteins.

Some combinations of amino acids are essential, some are not. Essential amino acids are the ones that cannot be made by your body and therefore must be obtained from your food. The foods that contain all of the essential amino acids in the proper proportions are good-quality proteins, or *complete proteins*. Animal sources of protein—meat, fish, fowl, eggs, and dairy products—are complete, with the exception of gelatin. Plant proteins, such as grains, beans, fruits, and vegetables, are incomplete, because they lack one or more of the essential amino acids or have insufficient amounts.

You can combine the "incomplete" plant proteins, such as beans, dried peas, lentils, nuts, and seeds, with complementary proteins, such as grains, potatoes, and corn, to form a complete source of protein. This is mandatory for vegetarians to insure adequate protein intake. Many people think there is no such thing as a fat vegetarian, but in fact, vegetarians often eat too much fat, since vegetable protein sources include seeds and nuts, which are high-fat foods. Eating too much food fat adds up to body fat, no matter whose calculator you use. If you are a non–red-meat vegetarian, you might consider eating only low-fat fish and fowl, instead of cheese, for protein, as you readjust your fat-to-muscle ratio. If you are a no-meat vegetarian, you might rely on bean and grain casseroles and soups. It is essential for you to get your protein daily and cut out the high-fat cheeses and nuts.

Red-meat-eaters must also be cautious of fat. The most common sources of protein might be meats and cheeses, but the best sources of energy and thermic responses are the lowest-fat meats and cheeses. In fact, meat is the major source of fat in the average American diet. If you are a red-meat addict, you would be wise to switch to the lower-fat fowl and fish and use red meat as a protein source no more than 3 times a week. In both of your diet phases, the meats have been preselected, so you won't have trouble staying low-fat with your meats, but at the end of your diet, be careful you don't fall back into the habit of eating large portions of meat, thinking you're getting good protein, when you are also getting too much fat.

It is a common misconception that you can eat a lot of protein without gaining weight. This way of thinking stems largely from the high-protein diets, which were supposedly good fat burners. When high-protein diets first came out, they were well received because people dropped weight fast. Actually, they were loosing weight simply because they were eating fewer overall calories, but eating a lot of protein felt like more eating, mostly because of the fat and bulky quality of meat. Even after the death scares from un-supervised high-protein diets, many people forgot that the false notions about high-protein diets came out of a decade that supported fast weight loss with high protein.

It's time to erase all the faulty information and start fresh. Not only does excess protein store as fat, but when you fill your diet primarily with protein, you are stripping away something else, and usually that's carbohydrates, your main brain food. When you eat a high-protein diet without protecting your daily dairy need, you are inviting calcium leeching from your bones and could wind up with bone deformities or osteoporosis. We'll talk more about that in the Dairy section, but to stay safe, remember, anything eaten to excess is a dangerous practice.

On the flip side of the coin, protein deficiencies are the last thing a dieter wants. When you do not have enough protein in your diet, your body will break down your muscle tissue in order to meet its protein needs and perform its basic functions. These muscle losses can be life-threatening if prolonged. Muscle is what you should gain on your diet, and this is as much a matter of life and health as a matter of fixing your fat-to-muscle ratio.

Another false belief about protein exists among athletes. Strenuous exercise does not require—and is not enhanced by—increased intake of protein. Rather, you need an increase in the total amount of calories you eat in the form of carbohydrates to meet the energy demands of higher levels of output through exercise.

How much protein is enough? Use the following formulas to determine your daily protein requirements for weight loss and weight maintenance.

Weight Loss:

(Your ideal body weight ÷ 2.2 [kilograms] × 1.2 (grams of protein per kilogram of body weight)

Maintenance:

(Your ideal body weight ÷ 2.2 [kilograms] × 0.8 (grams of protein per kilogram of body weight)

At an ideal body weight of 130 pounds, a person would need 71 grams of protein daily during weight loss and 47 grams of protein a day for long-term insurance of health.

Your ideal body weight is measured by the amount of lean body mass or muscle you have, and it can never be ideal unless you have enough muscle. So you can see that preserving your muscle is the single most important thing you can do on your diet, for your health and long-term weight maintenance.

Carbohydrates

Carbohydrates are your body's preferred source of energy and primary brain food. They are divided into two groups— simple (sugar) and complex (starches). Complex carbohydrates are actually long-chain simple sugars that are linked when you eat them and then split into simple sugars when your body digests and absorbs them. Why, then, are complex carbohydrates considered good and simple carbohydrates considered bad? The reason is found in the nutritional quality of the foods that contain these carbohydrates and your body's response to them.

First, complex carbohydrates are generally less-refined foods, and therefore are good sources of many other naturally occurring nutrients. Simple carbohydrates, or sugars, are usually very refined foods that have been stripped of their naturally occurring nutrients. Second, your body has a slower, more natural response to eating complex carbohydrates, gradually breaking down the longer chain to use for energy over prolonged periods—a longer thermic effect and longer energy boost.

Sugars exist in a very simple form, which stimulates a very rapid insulin response. They are absorbed easily and leave you feeling hungry sooner than if you ate a complex carbohydrate—shorter thermic response and shorter energy boost. People who eat high-sugar diets get short bursts of energy and big, tired letdowns. We won't go so far as to say that simple sugars are junk foods, because they do supply usable energy, but the energy is not first-quality, and for fat loss, the simple sugars are self-defeating, since they usually occur in foods that also contain a lot of fat.

The starch group of complex carbohydrates includes grains and grain products as well as starchy vegetables such as corn. They are excellent sources of B vitamins and fiber, especially when whole-grain varieties are eaten.

Vegetables and fruits are often mentioned together, because they have similar nutrient compositions. While fruit contains natural simple sugar that makes it sweet and higher in calories than vegetables, both fruits and vegetables provide healthy supplies of fiber and essential nutrients such as Vitamins A and C. In fact, one fresh grapefruit and one medium carrot will satisfy your total daily requirements for Vitamins A and C.

Dairy

Foods in the dairy group are good sources of protein and carbohydrates, the best source for Riboflavin (B^2) and the important mineral calcium.

Years ago people were warned away from calcium because they were consuming too much of it. Today, we find the situation has reversed. More and more studies are showing serious calcium deficiencies in Americans, which can lead to bone deterioration and cause heart disease, hypertension, and high blood pressure. Calcium deficiencies affect everyone, but they are especially damaging in women.

A major health risk among American women is osteoporosis—a disorder caused by calcium being leeched from the bones. The entire skeletal frame becomes weak and brittle. While most of us begin to lose bone density after the age of 25, hormonal changes in menopause accelerate the process. By age 60, 1 out of 4 American women have osteoporosis, causing pain, loss of height, spinal deformity, and spontaneous fractures caused by prolonged calcium deficiency.

Calcium leeching begins when your diet is too low in calcium and your body begins to release the calcium from your bones and teeth. Normally, your bones can store enough calcium to remedy this deficiency, but when your diet does not contain enough calcium to replace the bone losses, the lost calcium is not restored to your bones.

Calcium in your bloodstream can gather as spurs in your heels or joints. These spurs usually occur after an injury to the area, as for example heel spurs from jogging on hard ground or elbow spurs from tennis injuries. Calcium deposits can also be triggered by inflammation from arthritis, and unfortunately, calcium leeching from the bones is increased when steroids are taken for relief of arthritic pain. Athletes who take steroids invite calcium leeching and the resulting bone deterioration, especially if there diets are also high in protein.

High-protein diets can prevent calcium absorption. Studies have shown that osteoporosis runs high in people with high-protein diets in which the protein comes from animal sources that are also high in fat. Vegetarian women who eat no meat-fat proteins show less bone loss than meat-eating women as they age. Diets that are too high in protein have been linked to doubling bone loss at any age.

Before your body can use calcium, it must interact with all of the other vitamins and minerals: A, B-complex, C, D, magnesium, phosphorus, and potassium. Dieters who cut calories without concern for their nutrients face calcium deficiency and later-life bone deterioration.

On the plus side, exercise increases calcium absorption, all the more reason to exercise during your diet. The best absorption of calcium takes place when you take your calcium in smaller amounts over the course of a day rather than all at once in a large glass of milk. This is one of the reasons that we spread your calcium throughout your day. We want you to absorb it. Low-fat milk and dairy products are the preferred sources.

Calcium is a critical daily need. The recommended dose for adults is 800 milligrams per day, but many nutritionists are suggesting up to 1,000 milligrams per day, depending on your degree of risk for osteoporosis. Check with your doctor for the right dose and source of calcium for you if you are allergic to lactose in dairy products.

Fats

Ten little french fries have 10 big grams of fat.

You need some fat in your body for insulation, support, and protection of your organs, and to act as a carrier for the fat-soluble vitamins A, D, E, and K, aiding in their absorption.

Fat supplies essential fatty acids, including linoleic acid, which is needed for proper growth in children, to maintain cell membranes and regulate cholesterol metabolism, and to prevent drying and flaking of the skin. But how much fat do you need?

Studies show that 1 tablespoon of corn oil—rich in linoleic acid—provides all the essential fat needed by most people.

The average American derives 40–45 percent of his or her calories from fat. In fat intake studies of 35- to 40-year-olds, only 13 percent of the males and 17 percent of the females had a fat intake of less than 35 percent of their total calories. Over a third had a fat intake providing 45 percent or more of their total calories.

There are three kinds of fats in food: saturated, monosaturated, and polyunsaturated. Among these, saturated fats are the ones to avoid. Saturated fat is considered bad fat because it raises your blood cholesterol. Nature has made the saturated fats pretty simple to detect: They exist primarily in animal foods. Cheese, ice cream, butter, whole milk, and meats are saturated. Of all the vegetables, only coconut and palm are highly saturated—and watch out for them in coffee whiteners and processed foods. In fruits, only the avocado is saturated, so guacamole lovers are getting a lot of fat. If you see a food label stating that the product contains monosaturated fat, you are in neutral territory, since monosaturated fats do not increase blood cholesterol. But why take chances? If you must eat fat, eat polyunsaturated. These are the preferred fats, since they lower your blood cholesterol.

Dietary trends over the last decade indicate that our total intake of calories is down, so why are we still fat? Our fat consumption is up. We are eating more fat packed into fewer calories.

• We may not be eating more ice cream, but we are

choosing higher-quality ice cream with less air whipped in. *More fat.*

- We are still getting the major part of our fat from meats, and prime cuts are making a comeback. What are the primes highest in? *Fat.*
- We are eating less butter and lard than our ancestors, but we are increasing our consumption of fatty oils. We use more margarine, shortening, and salad and cooking oils. These are the sneaky fats we can slip into a sauce without noticing. Among the oils, the highest in saturated fats—palm and palm kernel—are our second-favorite oils. Coconut—also highly saturated—is our third-favorite oil. Soy, on the other hand, is polyunsaturated, and we are eating soy, but safflower (the most polyunsaturated) rarely makes the chart, and corn (more polyunsaturated than soy) is down on our list of favorites.
- We are eating more salads, but choosing high-fat varieties soaked in oils and using salad dressings as if they had no fat or calories, spooning in oversized amounts of fat.

Earlier, we mentioned that fat may increase your desire for sweets, and dietary trends support this finding. In the studies in which fat consumption is up, so is the switch from complex carbohydrates to simple ones, to eating more sugars.

Fat is insidious: The way it reacts in your system, it would seem that fat's only desire is to get more fat. You may think, at first, that cutting fat is going to be the most difficult challenge of your life. And it might be, but the results will be dynamic. You will feel a cleaner, lighter system in the absence of excess *fat.* You will begin to notice the flavor and subtle tastes of other foods that you may not have appreciated before, because your taste buds were blunted by your desire for the taste and texture of fat.

When you begin to withdraw from fat, you will suddenly appreciate how heavy fat is when you eat it. How slug-

gish you feel after a high-fat meal. How greasy it makes
your palate. By the time you start to feel deprived of fat,
you will already have made great strides in removing its
hold over your life. Then you will be able to choose—without abusing—*FAT*.

EMERGENCY THERMIC BOOSTERS

During the day, you may be *cued* to eat by an emotional
upset, a frustrating experience, too much stress, or any
number of *trigger* situations that could send you to food.

At those times, when you reach for food, what do you
usually reach for? High-fat or high-sweet. A candy bar is a
boost, but it's a quick hit that drops you just as quickly,
and it's high in fat. A cheese snack is a quick sense of comfort because it's high-fat, but it also leaves you sluggish
and nonthermic! These cues are grabbers that can break
your diet.

Next time you reach for a booster, switch your bad habits
for good ones and reach for foods that will keep your thermic
switch high.

Burn	Bomb
Crisp vegetables with dressed-up yogurt dips*	Chips with sour cream dips
Fruitsicles*	Ice Cream
Fruit and yogurt parfait*	Cheesecake
Frozen berry buds—strawberries, blueberries, raspberries*	Candy bar
Microwave or air-popped popcorn	Pretzels, nuts
Cracker nips with fruit spread*	Cookies
Fruit exotics—mango, pineapple, papaya, kiwi*	Chocolate
Thermic pizza*	Regular pizza

Creative potato skins*	Submarines
Yogurt spreads*	Cream cheese spreads
Fish-and-veggie roll-ups*	Fishburgers and hamburgers
Stir-fry delights*	Sandwiches
Spritzers*	Diet sodas
Fruit Frappés*	Milkshakes
Spicy Mary*	Bloody Mary
Mixed bag*	Nut mixes

*Recipes follow

Yogurt dips and spreads: See Recipes, Ch. 13.

Fruitsicles: Make ice pops of sweet fruits by pouring your favorite juice into an ice-cube tray. When they freeze, pop one out and enjoy it. You can keep a supply of pops around for half the price of supermarket pops.

Fruit and yogurt parfait: See Recipes, Ch. 13.

Frozen berry buds: Keep a supply of fruit buds in the freezer to perk up your taste sensations. Wash a pint of your favorite berries or grapes, place in a storage bag in the freezer. In about 2 hours, you have pick-me-ups ready to eat. Watch out for grapes and don't eat too many! They're a higher-concentrated sweet.

Cracker nips with fruit spreads: Crackers alone can be dry and unappealing. But topped with fruit slices and spreads, they become moist, tasty boosters. A cracker topped with apple slices and a dab of low-fat cottage cheese and sprinkled with cinnamon makes you think you're eating fruit danish.

Fruit exotics: Peel, cut into chunks, and refrigerate your favorite fruits. They'll be ready when you need something sweet.

Thermic pizza: Split an English muffin or pita loaf, top with a tablespoon of tomato sauce and spread. Sprinkle with basil and oregano. If you must have cheese, use a half ounce of low-fat mozzarella. Pop in toaster oven or broil. (No more than one muffin for a boost!)

Creative potato skins: Bake a few potatoes and scrape out

the insides (save for mashed potatoes for the family). Slice and stuff with veggies, chopped fine, steamed, or stir-fried, and mix with low-fat cottage cheese or yogurt spreads with spices. Experiment for variety! Store in the refrigerator or freeze to have available for dinner appetizers or snacks.

Fish and veggie roll-ups: Lightly steam your favorite vegetables, finely chopped (asparagus, broccoli, or cauliflower, which has the consistency of cheese when shredded and heated, or a mix of vegetables). Take a white, thin fish like flounder, sole, or scrod. Roll your vegetables into the fish and seal with a toothpick. Sprinkle with lemon and salt and bake at 325 degrees for 10–12 minutes. You can also use whole stalks of asparagus, lightly steamed.

Stir-fry delights: Mix your vegetables, add your chicken or fish, and stir-fry into great mixes with tomato sauce or light soysauce or ginger for a bit of spice. Experiment for your favorite combinations. You can stir-fry eggplant parmesan in a snap with chopped eggplant, onions, peppers, mushrooms, and cauliflower in a tomato sauce mix. Lightly sprinkle with cheese but keep it low-fat mozzarella and light. You can stir-fry vegetable stews and freeze them.

Spritzers: Mix seltzer water with a wedge of lime or lemon, or with 1–2 ounces of your favorite fruit juice. Add lots of ice for a refreshing pickup that beats a diet soda.

Fruit frappés: In a blender, pour 8 ounces of low-fat or skim milk, a cup of strawberries, half a banana, or a peeled peach. Toss in ice cubes (add a touch of saccharine or Nutrasweet if necessary). The result is a great shake that's low-fat and healthy.

Spicy Marys: Instead of the alcohol version, make a Spicy Mary with tomato juice, horseradish, Rose's lime juice, tobasco, pepper, and Worcestershire sauce. Don't forget the celery stick or cucumber stalk for pizzazz!

Mixed bag: Instead of fancy nut mixes with high-fat nuts, carry this mix in your attaché case or bag: Unsweetened Miniwheats, raisins, and Cheerios toasted in the oven, cooled, and carried in a booster bag.

Remember: When you reach for a booster or snack, consider it one of your daily *Hotplate* servings and account for it. If it's a small booster like a berry bud, you don't have to count it. If it's thermic pizza or stir-fry, count it.

RELIEF: EXERCISES FOR RELAXATION, TENSION RELEASE, AND STRESS REDUCTION

You can practice *relief* in stages, or steps, moving on to the second step after you are comfortable with the first step. Your goal is to become comfortable enough to move through the entire program in one session. Don't worry if you don't feel relief right away. Continue to practice the techniques and go through the motions. Eventually relief will begin to flow.

Find a quiet place where you can be alone without interruption. If you can, unplug the phone. Sit in a soft chair with your feet touching the floor and your hands loose in your lap or lying loosely on the arms of the chair. We don't recommend lying down, since you could fall asleep, and we want you to experience the full benefits of relief.

Rhythmic Breathing

Close your eyes and clear your mind. If your mind wanders or nags you about things you left undone, let the thoughts flow right through your mind. If the thoughts nag too much, imagine them as clouds of words that are passing out of your mind. Let the thoughts go.

Inhale slowly to the count of 3. Hold your breath for 3 counts, then exhale slowly to the count of 3.

Repeat this cycle of breathing 5 or 6 times until the rhythm becomes natural and easy. Each time you inhale, feel the oxygen filling your entire body, and each time you exhale, feel the tension flowing out with your breath.

Continue to breathe deeply and rhythmically, going deeper and deeper into relaxation with each breath. As you continue to breathe rhythmically, going deeper and deeper, your body will begin to feel heavier and heavier.

Let yourself feel heavier and heavier.

Full Body Relief

Start at your toes and relieve every part of your body by letting go with each muscle group. Feel the oxygen flowing through your body as you breathe, and feel tension letting go as you relieve each part of your body.

Toes: Talk to yourself with a soothing inner voice or a soft whisper. Say: "All of the muscles in my toes are letting go. My toes feel limp and heavy. My toes are loose, limp, and heavy. Tension is flowing out of my toes. Relief is now moving up my body to my . . .

Feet: "All of the muscles in my feet are letting go. My feet feel limp and heavy. My feet are warm and heavy, sinking into the floor. Tension is flowing out of my feet. Relief is now moving up my body to my . . .

Ankles . . .

Continue to move upward, relieving each part of your body. Special areas for special relief are your stomach (especially helpful to prevent cramping and intestinal tension, which will help your digestion), your shoulders and neck (these are common areas for holding tension), and your jaws and facial muscles (pay special attention to your scalp).

Each time an area is relieved, imagine the tension flowing down your body and out your toes or fingers.

Continue to breathe rhythmically and enjoy the relaxed, floating experience of being free.

Creating Your Own Scene

In your relaxed state, create a very pleasant place, a calming scene, your own personal space. Visualize the place or vista where you can experience total serenity: an island beach with white sand and waves breaking, or a green forest with birds singing, or a mountain overlook with green valleys, or simply a chair at home by a crackling fire. Choose the scene that will give you the most peaceful feeling. This becomes your scene.

Imagine your scene. Breathe in and exhale deeply. Enjoy the scene as if you were really there. Put yourself there. Feel the scene around you. Feel the calm, peaceful feeling of being there and silently say to yourself "I, (say your own name), feel relieved."

Hold the scene and the peaceful feeling and tell yourself that tomorrow you will wake refreshed and revived, ready to face a new day—calm, confident, and feeling good about yourself.

The next day, when you feel tense, or are facing stress, or feel as if you are going to overeat, close your eyes, recall your scene, inhale deeply, and repeat "I, (say your own name), feel relieved."

You will then experience the calm, peaceful feeling to override your tension and stress.

Assertive Thinking

In your relaxed state, give yourself positive suggestions.

"I can handle pressure calmly and with control."

"I like myself. I respect my mind, body, health, and well-being."

"I can accomplish any goals I set for myself, without fear."

"I can achieve great things."

Being Lean

In your relaxed state, see yourself lean.

Feel firm and fit, and feel yourself lean.

Feel light, strong, and free.

Repeat: "I am lean, I am healthy. My body works in perfect harmony. My body is balanced. I am happy."

Unwinding at Night

Before bed, count backward from 3. Tell yourself that when you open your eyes you will feel totally relaxed and calm. Next, tell yourself you will fall into a peaceful, deep sleep. In the morning, you will awaken feeling more awake, confident, and ready to face the new day with energy.

FACING UP TO STRESS

Your face is the mirror of your emotions, a reflection of how you deal with stress. A stressed face is tense and tight. Frowns appear when you don't know they are there. Lines deepen over time and you can look older when you are young, angry when you think you're not. Toxins build in tense muscles and pockets of tension form.

Facial massage will help you unlock your tension and act as a mini–facelift to firm up your face while you are getting a fitter body. No skinny cheeks that dieters worry about. It's great for women and men.

Begin your tension release by practicing antistress facial massage for 5 or 10 minutes, 3 times per week.

Techniques

Loosening Up: Open your mouth wide, close it, and press. Close your eyelids tightly and press; then open your eyes wide. Release the tension in your neck by pressing your shoulders down and stretching your neck as you slowly move your head from side to side and around in a slow circle, first to the right, then to the left.

Pressure Points: A good way to unlock pockets of stress and stimulate blood flow is through your pressure points. This can be done at any time of day, in almost any setting.

Begin by sitting comfortably, letting your whole body relax. Then begin.

Temples Massage: Locate the hollows at the outside edges of your temples. Using your index and middle fingers on both hands, begin to press gently on both temples. Let your thumbs rest lightly on your cheeks. Make small circles with your index and middle fingers, circling toward your eyes. Continue this for 1 or 2 minutes. Breathe easily.

Eyebrows: Locate the pressure point above your nose between your eyebrows. Using your ring fingers, press toward the back of your head. Keep your fingers stationary and circle them on the pressure point for 2 to 3 minutes.

Nose: Locate the pressure points on your cheeks, close to your nostrils. Massage with small circles for 2 or 3 minutes, counterclockwise.

Jaws: Locate the sockets below your earlobes at the end of your jawbone. Use your middle fingers to massage counterclockwise.

Blood Flow: Locate the soft spot at the back of your head where your spinal cord meets the base of your skull, about 3 inches in from each ear. Use both hands with the first 3 fingers working in combination. Press and massage toward the ear.

Cheeks: Locate the hollow space below each cheekbone. Press your thumbs against the bone, applying pressure for 30 seconds.

REWARDS

In childhood, food is often used for reward or removed for punishment. Usually, the food is a high-fat or sweet one. Seldom will you hear a parent say, "You were terrific today. You get broccoli for a reward." It's usually apple pie with ice cream, or chocolate cake with whipped cream. When children treat themselves, it's usually with candy.

For punishment, children will be told "No dessert tonight." No candy. No ice cream. No apple pie.

As we grow, these habits become ingrained and we treat ourselves to sweets and fats to celebrate promotions, good fortune, relatives gathering for holidays, or friends getting together for parties, and when we feel bad about ourselves, we eat to reverse the punishment principle of childhood, when we weren't allowed to have that fat or sweet.

You want to begin to reward yourself with anything but food.

Choose your reward from the following list, and make up your own list as you go along. What you are celebrating is your low-fat status, your future health and well-being. Do it without food! Gradually, as you replace food rewards with nonfood rewards, you will be unlearning one of the major contributors to overweight as you age—eating patterns carried over from childhood.

Reward list:

1. Buy a Walkman for your walking program.
2. Order a balloongram to be sent to you.
3. Make something with your hands.
4. Plan an imaginary vacation to a faraway place. Check out brochures. Put a map of the world on your wall and plan a new vacation a week.
5. Send your laundry out this week.
6. Treat yourself to a body massage.
7. Go dancing.
8. Sit on a park bench and people-watch.
9. Make a pep-talk tape to play back to yourself.
10. Send yourself a singing telegram.
11. Go try on hats.
12. Buy yourself sexy underwear.
13. Start a collection of crazy socks.
14. Take a bubble bath.
15. Ask someone to pat you on the back and say, "Congratulations."
16. Paint a nightshirt, a T-shirt, or your sweatpants with funny sayings.
17. Go have a good laugh at a funny card shop.

18. Walk in a bird sanctuary.
19. Sign up for a charity walk-a-thon.
20. Get tickets to a concert or play.
21. Send a friend an admiring card. Post it to yourself.
22. Request a song for yourself on the radio.
23. Rent a VCR if you don't have one, and watch all the movies you missed.
24. Get dayglow shoelaces for your sneakers.
25. Make funny faces in the mirror and laugh at yourself.
26. Test drive Porsches.
27. Plant a garden or a windowbox of herbs.
28. Take a course you've been putting off (*not* cooking).
29. Give your collection of "bigger" clothes to Good Will.
30. Tell yourself you're great.

HOW TO HANDLE A DIET BREAKDOWN

We'd like to think you won't break your diet, and you'd like to think so too, but what if you do?

One day, you forget what you're doing and eat the way you used to eat. Or something happens to trigger emotional cues, and you wolf down half the kitchen. Or you wake in the middle of the night and sleep-eat your way through a week's worth of snacks. Or you do it intentionally. You know you are doing it.

Don't avoid it, deal with it.

A successful person isn't someone who never makes mistakes, but someone who knows how to deal with them. One of the biggest errors dieters make is not the break, but pretending it didn't happen, or giving up when it does. This time, do a little homework about your break and you'll learn a lot of valuable information about yourself.

Don't skip this step, or you won't be able to deal with another break.

Break Strategy

Write down everything you ate when you broke your diet and tally the fat and calories.

Now, practice "Relief." Or go for a half hour walk to clear your head.

Now, go back to your break record, and check it against the following break ratio:

- If you ate from 30 to 40 grams of fat, *forgive yourself* and go back to your diet, keeping an eye on your fat.
- If you ate from 50 to 60 grams of fat, *watch it,* but forgive yourself and go back to your diet, keeping a hard eye on your fat.
- If you ate 70 or more grams of fat, forgive yourself and *go back to Burn 1 for an extra week* to get back on track.

Don't eat less to compensate for your break.
Don't call yourself a failure.
Don't take a pill to try to numb your hunger.
Do some creative and critical thinking.

Ask yourself, what was the first food you ate? This food might have connections. Did you eat it often when you were a child? Why does it give you pleasure? What associations come to your mind about this food? Do you know the fat, carbohydrate, and protein content of this food? Is there a substitute for this food that would please you just as much, or enough to put up with it?

Remove this food from your environment and substitute the low-fat variety.

Now ask yourself, is there a food you *really wanted* but didn't have and ate this food instead of? In fact, did you eat twice as much of something else in order to make up for not having this food? What food comes to mind? Chocolate? Ice cream? Butter?

Now make a food diary.

This is a book that will always be handy and will be used exclusively for your thoughts about food. Write down the foods you went for, the foods you wanted, and begin to make associations about them. Why you ate them, what time you ate them, whether a person was associated with them, how you felt, what your mood was, whether you could resist them. Then do a quick analysis of the nutrient content of these foods. Do some calculations. For every dish of ice cream, you could have how many servings of sherbet? How many popsicles? How many vegetables with low-cal dip? How much air-popped popcorn? Don't eat any of these things, simply check out the differences between your *go-for* foods and ones you don't go for.

Draw pictures of the food, do cartoons of something breaking the power of the food, and let yourself have a little fun in your Food Diary. Whatever comes to mind, write it down.

The next time you feel an urge coming on to break your diet, reach for your diary and read about the foods you went for on your last break. Then write about your urge to break. Go for a walk to clear your head.

Don't do any of this unless you break your diet. Save this strategy for the time of your break, because that is the time you'll learn the most about yourself.

Break Followup

Mark the break day on your diet calendar.

Make a break list to tack to the refrigerator, called "Break Tested."

"Break Tested" Checklist

List a number of alternatives you can use to get through your urge to break. Check off a technique each time you use it successfully to get past your "break" phase.

- Chew a piece of sugarless gum.
- Pop a frozen berry into your mouth and let it defrost its sweetness.

- Set a timer for 20 minutes (when hunger abates) and go for a walk.
- Splash cold water on your face. Or dunk your face into a sinkful of cool water and exhale through your nose while thinking that you are exhaling the urge.
- Take a bath and sip lemon water.
- Do relaxation exercises.
- Remind yourself you are breaking an addiction to fat and exercise instead.

These tricks are behavior substitutes to get you through the tough times. You may find you check off one more than others. In that case, you have a good habit that works for you.

If another one works, then you'll have two good behavior substitutes that work for you. Get as many as you can. These will carry you through life. However, if you find that the one you choose isn't working, go back to one that does, or run through the whole list to avoid a break. Or invent a new one on the spot and add it to your list.

TEN

MAINTENANCE: KEEPING YOUR LOW-FAT STATUS FOR LIFE

The following table will show you the recommended fat ceiling for low-fat maintenance for life. This will give you a good guideline for the fat maximum that will keep you healthy and prevent your fat from coming back.

As you can see, you are allowed more fat in maintenance when you have adjusted your body ratio of fat to muscle. At this point, your tolerance for fat will have dropped. You can use Burn 2 as a foundation, adding more carbohydrates and protein and a few more fats if you need them, but you must keep an eye on your *fat max* ceiling. You will also be eating more calories at maintenance, and the best thermic sources are still carbohydrates and low-fat proteins.

At maintenance, you need a higher calorie maximum to balance your input and output, but the skills you learned in dieting must carry over. You continue to eat low-fat and continue to exercise, but at maintenance you may find you can exercise 3 times a week and maintain your lower-fat status.

Recommended Dietary Fat Maximum for Maintenance

Projected Body Weight	Recommended Daily Fat Grams*	Approximate Maintenance Calories
90–100 lbs	33–40 grams	1,500 calories
100–110 lbs	33–46 grams	1,500–1,650 calories
110–120 lbs	37–50 grams	1,650–1,800 calories
120–140 lbs	40–58 grams	1,800–2,100 calories
140–160 lbs	40–58 grams	2,100–2,400 calories
160–180 lbs	40–58 grams	2,400–2,700 calories
180–200 lbs	40–58 grams	2,700–3,000 calories

*Fat grams listed are based on the recommended 20–25 percent of total calories as fat.

HOW TO EAT FOR MAINTENANCE

Here's a sure-fire way to stay lean and keep burning when you hit maintenance. You'll be using two tools: your Daily Diet Tray and Food Lists for Burn 2; your Fat Gram Counter and Fat Gram Goals for Maintenance.

Using your Burn 2 Daily Diet Tray and Food Lists will give you the best thermic foundation for building a higher-calorie, nutritious diet at maintenance.

Step 1: Add the foods in the following table to your Daily Diet Tray.

Guidelines

Calorie Level	New Food Plan	Foods Added
1,500 calories	2 servings protein 3 servings dairy 5 servings starches 5 servings vegetables 3 servings fruit 2 servings fat	1 dairy, 1 starch, 1 vegetable, 1 fat
1,650 calories	3 servings protein 3 servings dairy	Above plus 1 protein

Calorie Level	New Food Plan	Foods Added
	5 servings starches 5 servings vegetables 3 servings fruit 2 servings fat	
1,800 calories	3 servings protein 3 servings dairy 6 servings starch 5 servings vegetables 4 servings fruit 3 servings fat	Above plus 1 starch, 1 fruit, 1 fat
2,100 calories	3 servings protein 4 servings dairy 7 servings starch 6 servings vegetables 5 servings fruit 3 servings fat	Above plus 1 dairy, 1 fruit, 1 vegetable, 1 starch
2,400–3,000 calories	At this calorie level, most people can afford to include a sweet treat or two in their daily diet. This is acceptable as long as you don't compromise your power-packed diet base in favor of calorie-dense goodies. You also *must* keep your fat level down, within the limits defined for your calorie range.	

COUNTING YOUR DAILY FAT GRAMS

Refer to the appendix of foods in the back of the book. This is your Fat-Gram Counter. You'll notice that we rated over 300 foods. Included are the serving sizes, calories-per-serving, fat grams per serving, percent of total calories as fat, and a fat rating: No-Fat, Low-Fat, Medium-Fat, High-Fat.

Throughout your fat loss diet on Burn 1 and Burn 2, you omitted foods in the High-Fat range, except for 1 serving of fat during Burn 2. This had a twofold purpose: You broke your addiction to high-fat foods and high-fat cooking and you packed the most possible nutrients into a calorie-restricted diet to maximize your body fat loss.

Now that you've reduced your percent of body fat, reached your goal size, and maximized your burning power, you're able to maintain your weight while eating more calories. This allows you more flexibility and variety in your food choices—within fat limits.

Once you've built the framework of your maintenance program, using the guidelines for your fat max for life, start keeping track of your Fat Grams to insure an optimal thermic burn from your food and to help keep your body composition in its proper proportions.

Before you go for greasy, high-fat potato chips or high-fat cheese, ask yourself: "Can I afford the fat density of one food in my total daily calorie limit?"

Study the food lists in the Fat-Gram Counter to familiarize yourself with the fat ratings of various foods. Scan the list, using the rating system to get a good idea of the worst fat culprits.

Count your fat grams daily as a sure-fire way to keep your weight and fat in check.

FAIL-SAFE MAINTENANCE

If you keep an eye on your fat habits and eat more thermically, with exercise as a regular routine, you will maintain your low-fat status without difficulty.

However, if you find yourself slipping into old patterns of eating more and exercising less, here's what to do:

Set a weight maximum that spells danger!

Pick two weights that will dictate different behaviors.

If you reach a weight *5 pounds above* your ideal size, go back to Burn 2 for 1 or 2 weeks to regain control.

If you reach a weight *10 pounds above* your ideal size, go back to Burn 1 for 2 weeks.

Both of your thermic diets are fail-safe maintenance plans that you can rely on for life.

Remember: One bout of overeating does not make you fat; what does is *repeated* overeating and inactivity.

When you catch your bad habits before they get out of hand, you'll find it easy to keep your fat-to-muscle ratio in line for life. In addition to looking and feeling younger and stronger, you will be setting yourself up for ease, not disease.

Maintenance is not a state of total fat avoidance (although this wouldn't be a bad idea); it's making the best food decisions and coupling that with a regular exercise routine for positive self-enhancement.

If you can't find a particular brand name food on the Fat-Gram Counter in the back of the book, look up a similar generic counterpart instead and use that food's values. If you can't find a generic equivalent, check the nutrition information on the food's label, if available.

If you are creating a new recipe or figuring the fat in an old favorite, simply find the fat content of each food and add the fat grams for the total.

You now have the tools to keep your new body burning fat at peak levels for life!

Congratulations!

You earned it.

You have the power to achieve great things.

You have a right to be proud of yourself.

ELEVEN

BURN 1 MENUS

Please note: Your menus use your Daily Diet Tray formula, not your Hotplate formula. Therefore, when you use a menu, use the whole day.

BURN 1 DAY 1	FOOD GROUPS:

Breakfast:

Swiss Muesli*	1 serving starch
[Coffee or tea]	1 serving fruit
	½ serving dairy

Lunch:

3 oz cold chicken with Yakitori Marinade*	1 serving protein
½ c brown rice	1 serving starch
Small salad	2 servings vegetables
1 c snow peas	
Fresh peach	1 serving fruit
½ c plain, low-fat yogurt	½ serving dairy

Dinner:

3 oz Fish (haddock) Steamed with White Wine and Tarragon*	1 serving protein
4 new potatoes	2 servings starch
1 c steamed carrots	2 servings vegetables

*An asterisk indicates that this recipe appears in Chapter 13.

| Fresh orange | 1 serving fruit |
| 1 c skim milk | 1 serving dairy |

BURN 1 DAY 2

FOOD GROUPS:

Breakfast:

½ toasted bagel	1 serving starch
1 c melon cubes with blueberries	2 servings fruit
1 c plain, low-fat yogurt	1 serving dairy

Lunch:

Mixed Vegetable Pita*	1 serving protein
½ c grapefruit and kiwi compote	1 serving vegetable
	1 serving starch
	1 serving fruit

Dinner:

3 oz Chicken Caccia-tore*	1 serving protein
1 c angel hair pasta	1 serving vegetable
Fresh zucchini spears	2 servings starch
Salad	2 servings vegetables
1 c skim milk	1 serving dairy

BURN 1 DAY 3

FOOD GROUPS:

Breakfast:

1 c cold cereal	1 serving starch
1 c skim milk	1 serving dairy
½ c grapefruit juice	1 serving fruit

Lunch:

Black Bean Soup*	1 serving protein
Large tossed salad with Herb Dressing*	2 servings vegetables
2 bread sticks	1 serving starch

Lunch (cont.):

½ c fresh berries	1 serving fruit
½ c low-fat vanilla yogurt	1 serving dairy

Dinner:

3 oz Turkey Scallopini*	1 serving protein
1 baked potato with dollop yogurt	2 servings starch
½ c broccoli spears with lemon	2 servings vegetables
Sliced tomato	
Apple Cobbler*	1 serving fruit

BURN 1 DAY 4   FOOD GROUPS:

Breakfast:

1 slice pumpernickel bread	1 serving starch
½ c fresh berries	1 serving fruit
1 c plain low-fat yogurt	1 serving dairy

Lunch:

Stuffed tomato with Vegetable Tuna Salad*	1 serving protein 1 serving vegetable
2 garlic bread sticks	1 serving starch
1 c fresh strawberries	1 serving fruit
1 c skim milk	1 serving dairy

Dinner:

1 c spinach fettucini with Quick and Easy No-Fat Tomato Sauce*	2 servings starch 1 serving vegetable
½ c steamed yellow squash with scallions	2 servings vegetables

Tossed salad with ⅔ c kidney beans and Country Dressing*	1 serving protein
¼ cantaloupe wedge	1 serving fruit

BURN 1 DAY 5   FOOD GROUPS:

Breakfast:

1 slice rye bread with Hungarian Cheese Spread*	1 serving starch 1 serving dairy
½ c orange juice	1 serving fruit

Lunch:

1 c cold pasta and vegetable salad with Country Dressing*	2 servings starch 1 serving vegetable
3 oz crab meat	1 serving protein
Leaf lettuce	1 serving vegetable
Fresh seasonal fruit	1 serving fruit
½ c plain low-fat yogurt	½ serving dairy

Dinner:

3 oz Scallops with Scallions and White Wine*	1 serving protein
½ c Brown Rice Pilaf*	1 serving starch
½ c broccoli	2 servings vegetables
Romaine tossed with lemon juice and chives	
1 small apple, sliced	1 serving fruit
½ c plain low-fat yogurt	½ serving dairy

BURN 1 DAY 6   FOOD GROUPS:

Breakfast:
    ½ c hot oatmeal   1 serving starch
    Apple Cobbler*   1 serving fruit
    1 c skim milk   1 serving dairy

Lunch:
    3 oz turkey with dilled   1 serving protein
        cheese spread*   1 serving dairy
    1 slice black bread   1 serving starch
    Carrot sticks   1 serving vegetable
    Fresh fruit in season   1 serving fruit

Dinner:
    3 oz Chicken Breast   1 serving protein
        Baked with Herbs and
        Spinach*
    Baked potato with   2 servings starch
        dollop yogurt
    1 c string beans
    Large tossed salad   3 servings vegetables
    ½ c kiwi and raspberry   1 serving fruit
        mix

BURN 1 DAY 7   FOOD GROUPS:

Breakfast:
    1 toasted onion bagel   2 servings starch
    ¼ c low-fat cottage   ½ serving dairy
        cheese
    Fresh orange   1 serving fruit

Lunch:
    3 oz flaked tuna (water   1 serving protein
        packed)

Chilled asparagus with Herb Dressing*	2 servings vegetables
Tomato and cucumber chunks	
1 slice black bread	1 serving starch
2 slices fresh pineapple spears	1 serving fruit

Dinner:

Zucchini Lasagna*	1 serving dairy
	2 servings vegetables
1 slice Italian bread	1 serving starch
Tossed greens and	1 serving vegetable
Country Dressing*	1 serving protein
with ½ c garbanzos	
First Frost Compote*	1 serving fruit
	½ serving dairy

BURN 1 DAY 8 — FOOD GROUPS:

Breakfast:

1 c cold cereal	1 serving starch
1 c skim milk	1 serving dairy
¼ cantaloupe	1 serving fruit

Lunch:

Mixed Vegetable Pita*	1 serving protein
	1 serving vegetable
	1 serving starch
Tossed salad with	1 serving vegetable
Country Dressing*	
½ grapefruit	1 serving fruit

Dinner:

3 oz Fish (scrod) Steamed in White Wine and Tarragon*	1 serving protein

Dinner (cont.)

1 c green peas	2 servings starch
Marinated Tomatoes and Green Peppers*	2 servings vegetables
½ c applesauce mixed with 1 c plain low-fat yogurt and cinnamon	1 serving fruit 1 serving dairy

BURN 1 DAY 9   FOOD GROUPS:

Breakfast:

½ c orange juice	1 serving fruit
½ English muffin	1 serving starch
½ c Low-Fat Yogurt Spread*	1 serving dairy

Lunch:

Black Bean Soup*	1 serving protein
1 hard roll	2 servings starch
1 c green beans and tomatoes with Herb Dressing*	1 serving vegetable
2 pear halves	1 serving fruit
½ c low-fat vanilla yogurt	1 serving dairy

Dinner:

3 oz Chicken Breast Baked with Herbs and Spinach*	1 serving protein
½ c corn	1 serving starch
½ c brussels sprouts	1 serving vegetables
Large tossed salad with Herb Dressing*	2 servings vegetables
First Frost Compote*	1 serving fruit

Burn 1 Day 10

FOOD GROUPS:

Breakfast:
Swiss Muesli*

1 serving starch
1 serving fruit
½ serving dairy

Lunch:
Brown Rice Salad with
  Chicken and
  Vegetables*
Zucchini spears with
  Herb Dressing*
1 c strawberries
½ c plain low-fat yogurt

1 serving protein
1 serving vegetables
1 serving starch
1 serving vegetables

1 serving fruit
½ serving dairy

Dinner:
3 oz Scallops with
  Scallions and White
  Wine*
1 c broccoli
1 c green peas
½ c fresh pineapple
1 c plain low-fat yogurt

1 serving protein

2 servings vegetables
2 servings starch
1 serving fruit
1 serving dairy

BURN 1 DAY 11

FOOD GROUPS:

Breakfast:
1 c cold cereal
1 c skim milk
¼ cantaloupe

1 serving starch
1 serving dairy
1 serving fruit

Lunch:
Garbanzo Spread*
½ pita bread

1 serving protein
1 serving starch

Lunch (cont.):

Sliced tomato	2 servings vegetables
Cucumber spears	
½ banana	1 serving fruit
½ c low-fat vanilla yo-gurt	1 serving dairy

Dinner:

3 oz Turkey Scallopini*	1 serving protein
4 new potatoes	2 servings starch
½ c carrots	2 servings vegetables
½ c green beans	
Fresh fruit in season	1 serving fruit

BURN 1 DAY 12   FOOD GROUPS:

Breakfast:

½ toasted bagel	1 serving starch
1 c plain, low-fat yogurt	1 serving dairy
½ c berries	1 serving fruit

Lunch:

3 oz sliced chicken with dilled cheese spread	1 serving protein 1 serving dairy
1 slice pumpernickel bread	1 serving starch
Large tossed salad with Country Dressing*	2 servings vegetables
Fresh fruit in season	1 serving fruit

Dinner:

3 oz swordfish and vegetable kebobs with Yakitori Marinade*	1 serving protein 1 serving vegetable
1 c brown rice	2 servings starch
Tossed salad with Herb Dressing*	1 serving vegetable
Apple Cobbler*	1 serving fruit

BURN 1 DAY 13

FOOD GROUPS:

Breakfast:

½ toasted bagel	1 serving starch
½ c low-fat cottage cheese	1 serving dairy
½ c orange juice	1 serving fruit

Lunch:

3 oz flaked tuna (water packed)	1 serving protein
1 c cold pasta salad with vegetables and Country Dressing*	2 servings starch 2 servings vegetables
½ grapefruit	1 serving fruit

Dinner:

Chicken Cacciatore*	1 serving protein 1 serving vegetable
½ c white rice	1 serving starch
Romaine tossed with lemon juice and chives	1 serving vegetable
½ c fresh fruit cup	1 serving fruit
1 c skim milk	1 serving dairy

BURN 1 DAY 14

FOOD GROUPS:

Breakfast:

Swiss Muesli*	1 serving starch 1 serving fruit ½ serving dairy

Lunch:

Chef salad: 1 c lettuce	2 servings vegetables 1 serving protein

Lunch (cont.):

Tomato wedges	1 serving starch
Pepper rings	
Alfalfa sprouts	
Artichoke hearts	
1/3 c kidney beans	
1/4 c garbanzos	
1/2 c green peas	
with Country	
Dressing*	
1/4 c low-fat cottage	1/2 serving dairy
cheese	
1/2 pita bread	1 serving starch
Fresh fruit in season	1 serving fruit

Dinner:

3 oz broiled scrod with	1 serving protein
lemon and parsley	
1/2 c corn	1 serving starch
1 c beet salad with	2 servings vegetables
onion and Herb	
Dressing*	
1/2 c applesauce	1 serving fruit
1 c plain low-fat yogurt	1 serving dairy
and cinnamon	

TWELVE

Burn 2 Menus

BURN 2 DAY 1

FOOD GROUPS:

Breakfast:
½ English muffin   1 serving starch
½ c Low-Fat Yogurt   1 serving dairy
    Spread*
½ c fresh pineapple   1 serving fruit

Lunch:
Open-Faced Cheese   1 serving dairy
    Spread Sandwich*   1 serving starch
    with tomatoes and
    sprouts
Carrot sticks   2 servings vegetables
1 small apple, sliced   1 serving fruit

Dinner:
6 oz Chicken Breast   2 servings protein
    Baked with Herbs and
    Spinach*
1 c cauliflower   2 servings vegetables
Tossed salad
Acorn Squash New   2 servings starch
    England Style*
Dinner roll

*An asterisk indicates that this recipe appears in Chapter 13.

Dinner (cont.):

1 pat margarine	1 serving fat
½ c melon chunks and raspberries	1 serving fruit

BURN 2 DAY 2   FOOD GROUPS:

Breakfast:

1 c cold cereal	1 serving starch
1 c skim milk	1 serving dairy
½ c orange juice	1 serving fruit

Lunch:

6 oz Tangy Turkey Salad*	2 servings protein
	1 serving fruit
½ pita bread	1 serving starch
Tossed salad with Herb Dressing*	1 serving vegetable
½ c low-fat vanilla yogurt	1 serving dairy

Dinner:

1 c linguini with marinara sauce	2 servings starch
	1 serving vegetable
Tossed greens with Herb Dressing*	2 servings vegetables
Fresh plum	1 serving fruit

BURN 2 DAY 3   FOOD GROUPS:

Breakfast:

1 slice pumpernickel bread	1 serving starch
Hungarian Cheese Spread*	1 serving dairy
⅛ honeydew melon	1 serving fruit

Lunch:

Mixed Vegetable Pita*	1 serving protein
with Country	1 serving vegetable
Dressing*	1 serving starch
Marinated Tomatoes and	1 serving vegetable
Green Peppers*	
1 c fresh strawberries	1 serving fruit
½ c low-fat vanilla	1 serving dairy
yogurt	

Dinner:

3 oz baked chicken	1 serving protein
Baked potato skin	2 servings starch
stuffed with 2 c	2 servings vegetables
cauliflower, tomato,	
broccoli, mixed (see	
Creative Potato Skins,	
in Emergency Thermic	
Boosters)	
1 tsp margarine	1 serving fat
Apple Cobbler*	1 serving fruit

BURN 2 DAY 4   FOOD GROUPS:

Breakfast:

Swiss Muesli*	1 serving starch
	1 serving fruit
	½ serving dairy

Lunch:

Dilled Shrimp Salad*	1 serving protein
with raw vegetable	1 serving vegetable
garnish	
1 slice rye bread	1 serving starch
1 tsp margarine	1 serving fat
Tossed greens with Herb	1 serving vegetable
Dressing*	

Lunch (cont.):

Fresh orange	1 serving fruit
1 c skim milk	1 serving dairy

Dinner:

Turkey Cutlet Parmesan	1 serving protein
	½ serving dairy
½ c steamed summer	1 serving vegetable
squash with green	1 serving vegetable
onions	
1 c green peas	2 servings starch
½ c pineapple and kiwi	1 serving fruit
compote	

BURN 2 DAY 5

FOOD GROUPS:

Breakfast:

½ English muffin	1 serving starch
½ c low-fat cottage	1 serving dairy
cheese	
½ c orange juice	1 serving fruit

Lunch:

Garbanzo Spread*	1 serving protein
1 slice pumpernickel	1 serving starch
bread	
Cucumber chips	1 serving vegetable
½ c fresh fruit salad	1 serving fruit

Dinner:

Chicken Stew with	1 serving protein
Garden Vegetables*	1 serving vegetable
Tomato slices with basil	1 serving vegetable
and lemon	
1 baked potato	2 servings starch
1 tsp margarine	1 serving fat
Fresh seasonal fruit	1 serving fruit
1 c skim milk	1 serving dairy

BURN 2 DAY 6

FOOD GROUPS:

Breakfast:
½ toasted bagel
½ c Low-Fat Yogurt
   Spread*
½ c fresh blueberries

1 serving starch
1 serving dairy

1 serving fruit

Lunch:
Large spinach salad
   with tomatoes and
   sprouts, 1 oz shredded
   mozzarella cheese, and
   Country Dressing*
1 dinner roll
1 tsp margarine
Peach Crisp*

2 servings vegetables
1 serving dairy

1 serving starch
1 serving fat
1 serving fruit

Dinner:
6 oz Seafood with Wine
   Sauce* with ½ c
   broccoli
Baked tomato
1 c brown rice
Cucumber tossed with
   dill
First Frost Compote*

2 servings protein
1 serving vegetable

1 serving vegetable
2 servings starch
1 serving vegetable

1 serving fruit
½ serving dairy

BURN 2 DAY 7

FOOD GROUPS:

Breakfast:
½ c Cream of Wheat
   with cinnamon, ½
   sliced apple, and
   1 tbs raisins
1 c skim milk

1 serving starch
1 serving fruit

1 serving dairy

Lunch:

Brown Rice Salad with	1 serving protein
Chicken and	1 serving vegetable
Vegetables*	1 serving starch
Tossed greens with	1 serving vegetable
1 tbs salad dressing	1 serving fat
Fresh fruit in season	1 serving fruit

Dinner:

3 oz chicken and	1 serving protein
vegetable kebobs with	1 serving vegetable
Yakitori Marinade*	
1 baked potato	2 servings starch
½ c low-fat cottage	1 serving dairy
cheese with chives	
Garden greens with	1 serving vegetable
Herb Dressing*	
Fresh fruit in season	1 serving fruit

BURN 2 DAY 8

FOOD GROUPS:

Breakfast:

1 c cold cereal	1 serving starch
1 c skim milk	1 serving dairy
2 tbsp raisins	1 serving fruit

Lunch:

4 oz lean ground beef	2 servings protein
1 hamburger bun	2 servings starch
Sliced tomato	1 serving vegetable
Fresh orange	1 serving fruit

Dinner:

Zucchini Lasagna*	1 serving dairy
Tossed salad with	3 servings vegetables
Country Dressing*	

1 slice Italian bread	1 serving starch
1 tsp margarine	1 serving fat
½ c pineapple and kiwi compote	1 serving fruit

BURN 2 DAY 9

FOOD GROUPS:

Breakfast:

½ English muffin	1 serving starch
½ c low-fat vanilla yogurt	1 serving dairy
2 pear halves	1 serving fruit

Lunch:

Garbanzo Spread*	1 serving protein
1 slice pumpernickel bread	1 serving starch
Large spinach salad with Herb Dressing*	2 servings vegetables
½ oz mozzarella cheese	½ serving dairy
Fresh fruit in season	1 serving fruit

Dinner:

3 oz Chicken Breast Baked with Herbs and Spinach*	1 serving protein
½ c brown rice	1 serving starch
½ c green peas	1 serving starch
1 tsp margarine	1 serving fat
2 c cauliflower	2 servings vegetables
½ c plain low-fat yogurt	½ serving dairy
½ c blueberries	1 serving fruit

BURN 2 DAY 10   FOOD GROUPS:

Breakfast:

1 slice pumpernickel bread	1 serving starch
½ c low-fat cottage cheese	1 serving dairy
½ c applesauce with cinnamon	1 serving fruit

Lunch:

3 oz flaked tuna (water packed)	1 serving protein
1 c cold pasta, with:	2 servings starch
½ tomato, chopped	2 servings vegetables
Diced Onion	
½ c green pepper, chopped	
½ c green beans	
½ c carrot, chopped	
Country Dressing*	
½ c plain low-fat yogurt	½ serving dairy
½ c blueberries	1 serving fruit

Dinner:

3 oz Seafood with Wine Sauce*	1 serving protein
½ c broccoli	2 servings vegetables
Tossed salad	
½ corn on cob	1 serving starch
1 tsp margarine	1 serving fat
½ c plain low-fat yogurt	½ serving dairy
¼ cantaloupe, cubed	1 serving fruit

BURN 2 DAY 11

FOOD GROUPS:

Breakfast:
1 c cold cereal
1 c skim milk
½ banana

1 serving starch
1 serving dairy
1 serving fruit

Lunch:
Dilled Shrimp Salad*
Tossed salad with
   Country Dressing*
½ pita bread
Fresh fruit in season
½ c plain low-fat yogurt

1 serving protein
1 serving vegetable
1 serving vegetable
1 serving starch
1 serving fruit
½ serving dairy

Dinner:
3 oz Turkey Cutlet
   Parmesan

8 steamed asparagus
   spears
1 baked potato
1 tbsp sour cream
Fresh orange

1 serving protein
1 serving vegetable
½ serving dairy
1 serving vegetable

2 servings starch
1 serving fat
1 serving fruit

BURN 2 DAY 12

FOOD GROUPS:

Breakfast:
½ toasted bagel
½ c low-fat vanilla
   yogurt
½ banana

1 serving starch
1 serving dairy

1 serving fruit

Lunch:
Hungarian Cheese
   Spread*

1 serving dairy

Lunch (cont.)

1 pita bread	2 servings starch
Sliced tomato, cucumber, sprouts	2 servings vegetables
½ c pineapple	1 serving fruit

Dinner:

6 oz baked chicken with Yakitori Marinade*	2 servings protein
1 c green beans	2 servings vegetables
Tossed salad	
1 tbsp salad dressing	1 serving fat
½ c brown rice	1 serving starch
Fresh fruit in season	1 serving fruit

BURN 2 DAY 13   FOOD GROUPS:

Breakfast:

½ English muffin	1 serving starch
½ c low-fat cottage cheese	1 serving dairy
1 fresh peach	1 serving fruit

Lunch:

Tangy Turkey Salad*	1 serving protein
	½ serving fruit
½ pita bread	1 serving starch
Large tossed salad with Country Dressing*	2 servings vegetables
½ c plain low-fat yogurt	½ serving dairy
1 c strawberries	1 serving fruit

Dinner:

3 oz Scallops with Scallions and White Wine*	1 serving protein

1 c broccoli	2 servings vegetables
1 baked potato	2 servings starch
1 tsp margarine	1 serving fat
½ c skim milk	½ serving dairy
Fresh fruit in season	1 serving fruit

BURN 2 DAY 14

FOOD GROUPS:

Breakfast:

Swiss Muesli*	1 serving starch
	1 serving fruit
	½ serving dairy

Lunch:

3 oz sliced turkey	1 serving protein
½ oz mozzarella cheese	½ serving dairy
1 slice pumpernickel bread	1 serving starch
Sliced tomato and sprouts	2 servings vegetables
Cold asparagus with lemon	
¼ cantaloupe	1 serving fruit

Dinner:

2 oz rump roast	1 serving protein
4 new potatoes	2 servings starch
1 tsp margarine	1 serving fat
½ c carrots	2 servings vegetables
Tossed salad with Country Dressing*	
1 c skim milk	1 serving dairy
Fresh fruit in season	1 serving fruit

THIRTEEN

THERMIC BURN RECIPES: GOURMET DINING ON A THERMIC DIET

Following are 33 fabulous recipes for low-fat cooking—everything from entrees to cheese spreads, to salad dressings, to desserts. We've indicated the serving equivalents so you can mix and match them for your Hotplates. The recipes are listed in alphabetical order to make it easy for you to find any recipe that is called for in the menus in chapters 11 and 12.

Acorn Squash New England Style
(2 servings)

1 acorn squash
4 oz water pack pineapple (chunk or crushed)
¼ tsp cinnamon
½ cup apple juice
Vegetable spray

Wash and cut squash in half in the same direction as ribbing. Remove seeds. Spray a cookie sheet or shallow baking pan with vegetable spray. Place squash, cut side down, on cookie sheet. Bake at 350 degrees for 30 to 40 minutes or until squash is tender. Turn the cut side up and split each half into two halves. Top each wedge with 1 ounce of pineapple. Sprinkle with cinnamon and pour on 1 ounce of apple juice, letting juice soak into squash. Return to oven for 10 to 15 minutes to reheat and combine flavors.

For an interesting meal combination, let squash wedges cool to room temperature and top each with 1 serving of tangy turkey salad.

Serving Equivalents
1 serving starch
1 serving fruit

Apple Cobbler
(4 servings)

4 apples, peeled, cored, and sliced
¼ cup apple juice
1 tbsp lemon juice
Cinnamon and nutmeg to taste

Toss all ingredients. Place in shallow baking pan, cover with foil, and bake in 350-degree oven until apples are tender. Serve warm or chilled. Garnish with lemon or orange slices or a small dollop of plain yogurt. For added crunch, sprinkle 2 tablespoons of grapenuts over apples after baking.

Serving Equivalent
1 serving fruit

Black Bean Soup
(2 quarts; 6 servings)

1½ c dry black beans
1½ qt water
1 carrot, diced
1 onion, diced
1 potato, diced
2 celery stalks, diced
1 bay leaf
1 tsp oregano
¼ tsp savory
¼ tsp pepper
¼ tsp garlic powder
¼ c chopped fresh parsley
1 tbsp lemon juice

Soak beans overnight in enough water to cover. Combine soaked beans with water or chicken stock and all vegetables and seasonings. Simmer 1 hour. Add potatoes and simmer until potatoes are tender. Remove from heat. Add lemon juice and chopped parsley.

Serving Equivalent
1 serving protein

Brown Rice Pilaf
(1 serving)

¼ c brown rice, uncooked
Chicken Stock (see recipe)
Scallions or chives, chopped
Parsley and favorite herb, chopped

Simply follow any basic recipe for cooking brown rice, substituting chicken stock for water. Near the end of cooking

time, stir in a good handful of fresh chopped vegetables
and herbs.

Serving Equivalent
1 serving starch

Brown Rice Salad with Chicken and Vegetables
(1 serving)

½ c brown rice, cooked
3 oz cooked chicken, no skin
1 serving favorite vegetable (serving size varies according
  to vegetable selected)

Toss cooked brown rice and 3 ounces of cooked chicken
with your favorite vegetables. Use low-sodium soy sauce
and lemon juice to moisten and flavor the salad.

Options
For added flavor, add a half tablespoon of sesame oil and
count as fat serving.

Serving Equivalents
1 serving starch
1 serving protein
1 serving vegetable

Chicken Breast Baked with Herbs and Spinach
(1 serving)

1 skinless, boneless chicken breast
2 sprigs fresh dill

1 whole scallion
2 tomato slices (Italian plum tomatoes are best)
4 spinach leaves, washed
Pepper to taste
Aluminum foil
Vegetable spray

Spray fry pan with vegetable spray. Quickly brown chicken breast on both sides. Prepare a square of foil large enough to hold the chicken. Place chicken in foil, top with dill, scallion, tomato, and spinach. Sprinkle with pepper. Fold foil over to form neat package. Seal edges tightly. Place in baking pan and bake at 350 degrees for 15 to 20 minutes. Serve in foil pouch. When foil is opened, you will be greeted with a wonderful aromatic burst of steam.

Serving Equivalent
1 serving protein

Chicken Cacciatore in 15 Minutes
(1 serving)

1 boneless, skinless chicken breast
½ c no-fat or low-fat frozen tomato sauce (see recipe)
¼ c sliced fresh or canned mushrooms
¼ c chopped green pepper
Vegetable spray

Combine frozen sauce, mushrooms, and peppers in sauce pan and thaw over low heat, stirring often. When sauce has thawed, raise heat and simmer about 6 minutes to cook vegetables slightly. While sauce is cooking, spray a small fry pan with vegetable spray. Over medium heat, sauté the chicken breast until lightly browned on both sides. Pour hot sauce over chicken and simmer for 5 minutes or until breast is just cooked.

Remember: a boneless chicken breast will cook quickly. Do not overcook. Keep the chicken moist and tender and the vegetables crisp and crunchy.

Serving Equivalents
1 serving protein
1 serving vegetable

Chicken Stew with Garden Vegetables
(2 servings)

4 chicken pieces (one-eighths)
¼ c chopped onion, carrot, and celery
2 parsley sprigs
¼ tsp thyme
2 c Chicken Stock (see recipe)
1 small turnip diced and cooked
6–8 brussels sprouts
1 carrot, thick sliced
Vegetable spray

In heavy fry pan sprayed with vegetable spray, brown chicken pieces. Add the chopped vegetables, chicken stock, and seasonings, reserving the turnip, brussels sprouts, and sliced carrots. Cook till chicken is tender—35–40 minutes. Remove chicken, add turnip, sprouts, and carrot. Cook till tender. Add chicken to reheat. Serve in soup bowls with plenty of broth.

Serving Equivalents
1 serving protein
1 serving vegetable

Chicken Stock
(to make 3 quarts)

6 pounds of chicken parts (necks, backs, wings, etc.) or a
    large cut-up stewing chicken
3 large carrots peeled and sliced
1 onion peeled and cut in half, each half stuck with 1 clove
2 leeks, cleaned and chopped
1 stalk celery, cut in thirds
1 large clove garlic
6 parsley sprigs
1 tsp dry thyme
4½ qt cold water or enough to cover all ingredients

Place chicken parts in a large kettle and add water. Bring
to boil and skim off foam. Add all other ingredients and
reduce heat to simmer. Cook for at least 3 hours. Strain
stock through a fine strainer. Let cool and then refrigerate.
When stock has cooled, remove hardened fat from surface.
Divide stock into a number of different size containers and
freeze for future use. One good idea is to freeze an ice-cube
tray of stock in which to "sauté" vegetables rather than
using butter or oil. Also, use stock to cook pasta or potatoes.
After they are cooked, reduce this cooking liquid and use
as sauce. It will be full of flavor and thickened from starch
in the pasta or potato. Adding some fresh chopped parsley
and scallion can make a great side dish.

Country Dressing
(1 cup)

1 c buttermilk
1 tsp apple juice
1 tsp lemon juice
1 tsp green onion chives

1 tsp fresh dill
⅛ tsp allspice
⅛ tsp paprika
Pepper to taste

Combine all ingredients and chill.

Dilled Shrimp Salad
(1 serving)

20 medium shrimp
Favorite vegetable, chopped (celery, sprouts, frozen peas,
    cucumber, etc.)
Herb Dressing, to taste (see recipe)

Toss diced vegetable with herb dressing flavored with dill.
Mix in shrimp. Chill.

Options
Stuff shrimp salad into a pita bread or serve over a fresh
tossed salad.

Serving Equivalents
1 serving protein
1 serving vegetable

First Frost Compote
(1 serving)

1 medium apple
1 tbsp orange juice
3–4 tbsp plain low-fat yogurt

This is as easy as eating an apple. Simply grate a fresh,

unpeeled apple into orange juice. Stir in the yogurt to combine. Serve in a fancy glass garnished with a slice of orange.

Serving Equivalents
1 serving fruit
½ serving dairy

Fish Steamed with White Wine and Tarragon
(1 serving)

3 oz of fish (or chicken)
Dry white wine
Herb mixture

This is a quick, easy way to cook fish or chicken breasts. Simply place the fish or chicken in a shallow pan or fry pan. Add enough white wine to half cover the fish steak or fillet. Add your favorite herb mixture. Cover pan and steam until cooked. Remove fillet from pan and reduce cooking liquid to ⅓ to make a rich flavorful sauce. Pour over fish and serve.

This same method could be used for vegetables substituting chicken stock for the wine. Remember: Add your favorite herbs and spices.

Serving Equivalent
1 serving protein

Garbanzo Spread
(2 servings)

¼ c low-fat cottage cheese
1 tbsp lemon juice
1 c garbanzos (chick peas) (canned)

¼ tsp cumin
¼ tsp coriander
½ tsp garlic powder
¼ c diced cucumber
¼ c diced tomato

Place all ingredients except cucumber and tomato in food processor. Blend till smooth. Mix with diced cucumber and tomato. You can also add fresh green onion or dill for more flavor.

Serving Equivalent
1 serving protein

Herb Dressing
(1 cup)

½ c cider vinegar
4 tbsp apple juice
2 tbsp lemon juice
2 tbsp onion flakes
2 tbsp parsley flakes
½ tsp pepper
½ tsp tarragon
½ tsp oregano
½ tsp paprika

Mix ingredients and chill. Feel free to experiment with herb combinations. You may want to substitute fresh herbs and onions to provide a more exciting snap.

Hungarian Cheese Spread
(4 servings)

16 oz low-fat cottage cheese
1 tbsp finely chopped chives or 1½ tbsp freeze-dried chives

½ tsp garlic powder or to taste
1 tbsp paprika (use Hungarian if possible—the difference is incredible!)

Combine all ingredients, repack in plastic cottage cheese container and chill for at least one hour. This spread stores well and provides several days of quick meals. Use as a sandwich spread, vegetable dip, or baked potato accompaniment.

To vary this recipe, add such chopped vegetables as sweet red and green peppers, cucumbers, or tomatoes.

Serving Equivalent
1 serving dairy

Low-Fat Yogurt Spread
(4 servings)

16 oz plain low-fat yogurt
Chopped chives

Place 5 sturdy paper towels in the bottom of a colander and set on a mixing bowl. Spoon yogurt into colander and place the colander and the bowl in the refrigerator overnight (6–8 hours). The fluid in the yogurt will drain into the bowl leaving a condensed yogurt spread. Remove yogurt spread from colander and mix with chopped chives for a delicious sandwich spread or dip for vegetables.

Options
Instead of chives, mix yogurt spread with your favorite chopped vegetables or fresh herbs such as mint, parsley, or onion. You can even mix with chopped poached salmon for a wonderful fish spread. Even fruit goes great with yogurt spread.

Serving Equivalent
1 serving dairy

Marinated Tomatoes and Green Peppers
(2 servings)

1 fresh tomato
1 c sweet green pepper, chopped or in strips

Mix diced or wedged tomatoes with green peppers and
Herb Dressing (see recipe), lemon juice, or flavored vinegar.
Chill for two hours or overnight.

Serving Equivalent
1 serving vegetable

Mixed Vegetable Pita
(1 serving)

Leaf lettuce
⅓ c kidney beans
¼ c garbanzos (chick peas)
½ c small broccoli flowerettes
Chopped scallion
¼ c sliced zucchini
1 oz Herb Dressing (see recipe)
½ pita bread

Line the pita with lettuce leaf. Mix remaining ingredients
and stuff pita.

Serving Equivalents
1 serving protein
1 serving starch
1 serving vegetable

Open-Faced Cheese Spread Sandwiches

Combine Hungarian cheese spread with 1 slice of your favorite bread. Add any combination of fresh vegetables such
as leaf lettuce, sliced plum tomatoes, sprouts, cucumbers,
and scallions.

Serving Equivalents
1 serving dairy
1 serving starch
½ serving vegetable

Peach Crisp
(4 servings)

2 c water pack peaches sliced and drained
1 c grapenuts
¼ c raisins
Cinnamon and nutmeg to taste
¼ c plain low-fat yogurt

Combine all ingredients except yogurt in shallow baking
pan. Cover with foil. Bake in 350-degree oven until heated
and browned. Serve warm or chilled with yogurt topping.

Serving Equivalents
1 serving fruit
1 serving starch

Quick and Easy No-Fat Tomato Sauce
(1 cup = 1 serving)

2 qt crushed tomatoes (or try new chunky-style tomatoes)
1 c onions

2 tbsp chopped garlic (more if you like)
½ c chopped fresh parsley
¼ c chopped fresh basil
1 c dry red wine
Pepper to taste
Vegetable spray

In a covered, heavy-bottom sauce pan sprayed with vegetable spray, cook the onions, garlic, parsley, and basil over low heat until onions start to soften (6–8 minutes). Stir frequently to prevent sticking. Remove cover and add wine. Raise heat and simmer for 5 minutes. Add tomatoes, stir to combine, and cook slowly for 30–45 minutes. Sauce will reduce and thicken slightly. Add pepper to taste and serve. If making sauce for future use, freeze after cooling in several size containers. Plan some 1-, 2-, 4-, and 6-serving sizes so you can quickly pop a frozen sauce out of its container and right into a sauce pan. Heat slowly.

Note: Though dried herbs will be faster and easier, try to take the time and effort to use fresh. The benefits in flavor will make you happy some night when you come home from work tired and grumpy and ready to have a good meal.

To make this a more interesting low-fat sauce, add a quarter cup grated parmesan or romano cheese during the long cooking phase. (This is equivalent to 1 serving of high-fat dairy).

Serving Equivalent
1 serving vegetable

Ratatouille
(4 servings)

1 medium eggplant, cubed
1 small onion, chopped

1 small green or red pepper, strips
Fresh or dried seasonings, to taste, (parsley, garlic, basil,
   and black pepper)
½ lb fresh mushrooms, sliced
1 8-oz can plum tomatoes, crushed
Vegetable spray

Cover a no-stick pan with vegetable spray and heat. Add
eggplant, onion, pepper, and herbs to brown, stirring constantly to avoid sticking. Add mushrooms. Add crushed
tomatoes, lower heat and cover to simmer for 30–40 minutes.

Options
Serve over rice or pasta or use as a filler for a stuffed baked
potato. Add grated parmesan cheese or melt mozzarella
cheese for a total meal.

Serving Equivalent
1 serving vegetable

Scallops with Scallions and White Wine
(1 serving)

3 oz scallops (sea scallops are most succulent)
¼ c fresh scallions, thinly sliced
¼ c white wine
Vegetable spray
Pepper to taste
Lemon wedges

Spray a medium size fry pan with an even layer of vegetable
spray. Over high heat, quickly toss the scallions until the
green part starts to wilt slightly (about 4 minutes). Add the
scallops and the white wine. Cover, reduce heat to medium
and cook for 5–10 minutes, depending on size of the scal-

lops. Do not overcook. Scallops should not be firm or rubbery. Remove scallops and transfer to a warm plate. Raise the heat. Stirring constantly, reduce liquid in the pan to one-third. Pour over scallops. Season with pepper and lemon and enjoy.

Options
Try adding different herbs such as dill, parsley, basil, tarragon, garlic, or chives. These can work in combination (for example, chives, garlic, and tarragon) or as a single flavoring, if you prefer. Add a frozen vegetable such as broccoli, peas, or corn, or one of the new interesting vegetable mixes. Just make sure they are not frozen in butter sauce! Add the vegetable when you add the wine and scallops. Vegetables will cook in the same time as the scallops and you will have a wonderful meal in 10 minutes, all in the same pan!

Serving Equivalent
1 serving protein

Seafood with Wine Sauce
(1 serving)

3 oz favorite fish
¼ c fresh scallion, thinly sliced
¼ c white wine
Vegetable spray
Pepper to taste
Lemon wedges

Spray a medium size fry pan with an even layer of vegetable spray. Over high heat, quickly toss the scallions until the green part starts to wilt slightly (about 4 minutes). Add the fish and the wine. Cover, reduce heat to medium and cook for 5–10 minutes, depending on size of fish. Do not over-cook. Remove fish and transfer to a warm plate. Raise heat and, stirring constantly, reduce liquid in pan to one-third. Pour over fish. Season with pepper and lemon.

Options
Try a variety of fresh fish and add different herbs such as dill, parsley, basil, tarragon, garlic, or chives, or add them in combination if you prefer. Add a frozen vegetable when you add the fish, wine, and liquid for a wonderful meal in the same pan!

Serving Equivalent
1 serving protein

Strawberry Yogurt Pops
(8 servings)

16 oz low-fat vanilla yogurt
4 c fresh strawberries

Blend yogurt and strawberries in a blender or food pro-cessor. Fill a frozen pop tray with mixture and freeze for at least 4 hours.

Options
Substitute any of your favorite fresh fruits in season for a tasty refreshing treat. You can also spoon mixture into a parfait glass.

Serving Equivalents
1 serving dairy
½ serving fruit

Swiss Muesli Breakfast Treat
(2 servings)

1 c unsweetened Swiss familia cereal
1 apple, cored and diced
1/2 small banana, peeled and thinly sliced
1/8 c raisins
1 tbsp honey
1 c plain low-fat yogurt
1/4 tsp vanilla extract

Combine all ingredients. If Muesli looks dry, add small amount additional yogurt and serve in your best crystal goblets garnished with sprigs of fresh mint.

Serving Equivalents
1 serving starch
1 serving fruit
1/2 serving dairy

Tangy Turkey Salad
(2 servings)

5 oz cooked turkey, diced
3 oz celery
1 1/4 oz crushed pineapple (unsweetened)
2 oz plain low-fat yogurt
1 tbsp fresh parsley
1 scallion thinly sliced

Mix all ingredients and chill.

Serving Equivalents
1 serving protein
1/2 serving fruit

Turkey Cutlet Parmesan
(2 servings)

6 oz turkey cutlet (sliced breast available in the poultry case at market)
1 tbsp flour, seasoned with pepper
1 tbsp chopped garlic
1 tbsp chopped scallion
¼ c Chicken Stock (see recipe)
Vegetable spray
1 oz low-fat mozzarella cheese, shredded
2 c Quick and Easy Low-Fat Tomato Sauce (see recipe)

Dust the cutlets lightly with flour. Spray a fry pan with vegetable spray. Heat pan and quickly sauté the cutlets. After the cutlets have browned, place them in a shallow baking pan. Add the garlic, scallion, and chicken stock. Top with tomato sauce and shredded mozzarella cheese. Bake at 350 degrees until cheese is browned and bubbly.

Serving Equivalents
1 serving protein
½ serving dairy
1 serving vegetable

Turkey Scallopini
(2 servings)

6 oz turkey cutlet (sliced breast available in the poultry case at your market)
1 tbsp flour seasoned with pepper
1 tbsp chopped garlic
1 tbsp chopped scallions
2 tbsp chopped parsley
¼ c Chicken Stock (see recipe)
2 lemon slices
Vegetable spray

Dust the cutlets lightly with flour. Spray a fry pan with vegetable spray. Heat pan and quickly sauté the cutlets. After the cutlets have browned, remove them from the pan and keep warm. Raise the heat to high, add the garlic, scallions, parsley, and stock. Cook, stirring constantly, scraping up any brown bits in the pan. Reduce the liquid to one-third. Pour the sauce over the turkey and serve. Garnish each portion with 1 of the lemon slices and more chopped parsley.

Serving Equivalents
1 serving protein

Vegetable Tuna Salad
(1 serving)

3 oz water packed tuna, flaked
¼ cucumber, diced
¼ c alfalfa sprouts
¼ c sliced radish and zucchini, mixed
½ c chopped lettuce
¼ c diced firm tomato
1 tsp vinegar, flavored vinegar, lemon juice, or Herb Dressing (see recipe)

Mix all ingredients and enjoy as salad or fill a half pita for a great sandwich. You can vary the vegetables according to preference or season.

Serving Equivalents
1 serving protein
1 serving vegetable

Yakitori Marinade

1 c teriyaki sauce
1 oz sherry or sake

1 1-inch piece peeled fresh ginger
1 scallion cut in thirds
2 tbsp apple juice

Combine ingredients, pour over chicken, fish, filets or steaks, veal or beef, or seafood such as shrimp or scallops. Marinate for 1–2 hours, or overnight if you prefer a stronger flavor. Either bake, broil, or grill these foods quickly until just cooked. To add more interest, make kebobs combining both meat and fish (for example, chicken and shrimp) with fresh vegetables such as zucchini, onions, peppers, mushrooms, or cooked artichoke bottoms. Try these kebobs grilled on charcoal—they're great!

Zucchini Lasagna
(2 servings)

4 medium zucchini
1 c low-fat cottage cheese mixed with ½ tsp basil,
    ½ tsp black pepper, 1 tsp fresh parsley
2 c no-fat tomato sauce
1 c fresh mushrooms
Vegetable spray

Slice the zucchini lengthwise into quarter-inch-thick slices. Place zucchini on a cookie sheet sprayed with vegetable spray. Broil zucchini, turning frequently, until lightly brown. In a shallow baking pan, alternate layers of tomato sauce, zucchini slices, mushrooms, and cheese mixture, finishing with tomato sauce. Bake in 350-degree oven for 1 hour, or more if lasagna appears to be watery. Let lasagna cool for 15 minutes before cutting into squares. Serve with more tomato sauce if you like.

Serving Equivalents
1 serving dairy
2 servings vegetables

APPENDIX

FAT-GRAM COUNTER

This Fat-Gram Counter provides an alphabetical listing of over 300 foods.

Code:
- *Serving:* suggested serving size.
- *Calories:* supplied by carbohydrate, protein, and fat content.
- *Fat Grams:* amount of fat per serving.
- *Fat percentage:* percentage of total calories as fat.
- *Fat rating:* No = no fat per serving.
  - L = low-fat food.
  - M = medium-fat food.
  - H = high-fat food.
- Fat Ratings are based on percentage of total calories as fat.*

FACTS ABOUT YOUR FAT-GRAM COUNTER

The food servings in this counter are common household measurements so that you can conveniently portion your foods with confidence. Accurate portioning is essential, since food portions are directly related to calories. If your portion size goes up, so do your calories.

The portions of foods were also adjusted according to their fat content. The more fat the food contains, the smaller the portion size. This has a twofold purpose:

---

*Data compiled from current tables provided by U.S. Department of Agriculture.

- It enables you to control the fat content of your foods.
- It keeps you wise to cutting down on high-fat foods and filling up on low-fat ones.

Don't cheat yourself of nutritional balance. If you constantly select high-fat foods, you'll be jeopardizing your nutritional status by eating small quantities of fat-dense foods rather than large quantities of nutrient-dense ones.

The portion sizes for foods are based on *cooked* weight unless otherwise specified. Vegetables, however, can be portioned either cooked or raw.

Food	Serving	Calories	Fat Grams	Fat Per-centage	Fat Rating
Alfalfa sprouts	2 oz	20	0	0%	No
Almonds	½ oz	85	8	82	H
Anchovy	10 pc	70	4	50	M
Angelfood cake	1 pc	161	0	0	No
Apple, small	1	75	0	0	No
Apple butter	1 tbsp	33	0	0	No
Apple cider	4 oz	58	0	0	No
Apple juice	3 oz	45	0	0	No
Applesauce	½ c	50	0	0	No
Apricot, fresh	2	36	0	0	No
Artichoke hearts	4	30	0	0	No
Asparagus spears	8	27	0	0	No
Avocado	⅛	47	4	86	H
Bacon, slices	2 pc	86	8	84	H
Bagel (5″ dia)	½	160	0	0	No
Banana, small	½	40	0	0	No
Bass, cooked	3 oz	99	3	27	L
Beans, cooked:					
Baked	⅓ c	128	5	38	M
Black	⅔ c	150	2	12	L
Great Northern	⅔ c	141	1	5	L
Green/string/wax	1 c	31	0	0	No
Kidney	⅔ c	145	3	4	L
Lentils	⅔ c	141	—	0	No
Lima	⅔ c	126	0.5	4	L
Sprouts, fresh	½ c	19	0	0	No

Food	Serving	Calories	Fat Grams	Fat Percentage	Fat Rating
White	¼ c	153	1	6	L
Beef, cooked:					
Chuck, no fat	2 oz	141	8	50	M
Chuck, w/fat	1 oz	121	11	77	H
Corned	1 oz	105	9	74	H
Dried, creamed	¼ c	94	7	62	H
Ground					
(10% fat)	2 oz	124	6	46	M
(21% fat)	1 oz	78	6	69	H
Loin	2 oz	128	6	42	M
Round, no fat	3 oz	161	5	29	L
Round, w/fat	2 oz	148	9	53	M
Rump, no fat	2 oz	120	5	40	M
Rump, w/fat	1 oz	98	8	71	H
Steak, no fat	2 oz	128	6	42	M
Steak, w/fat	1 oz	132	8	82	H
Beets	½ c	31	0	0	No
Beverages:					
Carbonated sodas	12 oz	150	0	0	No
Tonic water	12 oz	113	0	0	No
Club soda	12 oz	0	0	0	No
Seltzer water	12 oz	0	0	0	No
Biscuit (2″ dia)	1	103	5	44	H
Blueberries, fresh	½ c	45	0	0	No
Bluefish, cooked	3 oz	135	4	3	L
Brazil nuts	2	60	6	90	H
Bread:					
Corn	1 sl	161	6	34	M
Crumbs	¼ c	98	1	10	L
English muffin	½	75	0	0	No
Pita (Syrian)	½ med	75	0	0	No
Sliced	1 sl	70	0	0	No
Sticks (5″)	2	76	0	0	No
Stuffing	¼ c	104	7	64	H
Broccoli	½ c	48	0	0	No
Brownie	1	97	7	58	H
Brussels sprouts	½ c	51	0	0	No

Food	Serving	Calories	Fat Grams	Fat Percentage	Fat Rating
Bulgur (wheat), cooked	½ c	114	0	0	No
Bun (hamburger, hot dog)	½	75	1	12	L
Butter	1 tsp	35	4	100	H
Cabbage	1 c	30	0	0	No
Cake:					
With icing	¹/₁₂ pie	362	14	36	M
Cupcake	1	185	7	34	M
Fruitcake (2 × 2 × ½)	1 pc	115	5	39	H
Pound (3 × 3 × ½)	1 pc	142	9	57	H
Sponge (2" wedge)	1 sl	146	3	18	M
Canadian bacon	2 oz	122	8	60	M
Candy:					
Caramels	3	150	5	30	M
Chocolate	1 oz	147	9	56	H
Fudge	1 oz	122	5	32	M
Hard	1 oz	110	0	0	No
Jelly beans	1 oz	100	0	0	No
Cantaloupe	¼	40	0	0	No
Carrots	½ c	48	0	0	No
Cashews	½ oz	80	7	74	H
Catsup	1 tbsp	15	0	0	No
Cauliflower	1 c	28	0	0	No
Celery	1 c	28	0	0	No
Cereal:					
Cooked	½ c	70	0	0	No
Granola	1 oz	130	4	28	M
Whole grain	1 c	100	0.5	5	L
Cheese:					
American	½ oz	55	4	73	H
Blue	½ oz	52	4	74	H
Brick	½ oz	52	4	74	H
Cheddar	½ oz	56	4	72	H
Cottage, low-fat	½ c	86	0.5	3	L
Cottage, regular	¼ c	60	5	36	H

Food	Serving	Calories	Fat Grams	Fat Percentage	Fat Rating
Imitation	1 oz	50	2	35	M
Mozzarella, low-fat	1 oz	80	5	56	M
Parmesan	½ oz	60	4	59	H
Processed Spread	½ oz	40	3	68	H
Swiss	½ oz	55	4	68	H
Cherries	½ c	41	0	0	No
Chicken:					
No skin, meat only	3 oz	141	3	18	L
With skin	2 oz	142	7	42	M
Drumstick	1	88	4	39	M
Salad	⅓ c	134	8	54	M
Thigh, fried	1 pc	250	18	65	H
Wing	1	82	5	49	M
Clams	15	168	2	9	L
Coconut, shredded	¼ c	70	7	91	H
Cod, cooked	3 oz	144	4	28	L
Coleslaw, with mayo	¼ c	44	4	82	H
Cookies, assorted	3	126	4	26	M
Corn chips	10	110	5	41	H
Corn on cob	½ ear	70	0	0	No
Corn kernels	½ c	70	0	0	No
Crab, deviled	¼ c	112	6	45	M
Crab meat	3 oz	86	2	22	L
Crackers:					
Butter	5	76	3	36	H
Cheese tidbits	10	40	3	68	H
Graham	1	55	1.5	24	M
Melba rounds	7	70	0.5	9	L
Oyster	20	60	6	10	L
Peanut butter/ cheese	3	103	5	44	H
Rice cakes	2	70	0	0	No
Saltines	5	62	1.5	22	M
Cranberry juice	2 oz	40	0	0	No

Food	Serving	Calories	Fat Grams	Fat Percentage	Fat Rating
Cranberry sauce	1/8 c	50	0	0	No
Cream:					
Cheese	1 tbsp	52	5	96	H
Half & half	1 tbsp	20	2	90	H
Sour	1 tbsp	25	3	90	H
Whip	1 tbsp	53	6	95	H
Croissant, plain (5″ dia)	1	275	13	43	H
Cucumber	1	25	0	0	No
Custard	1/2 c	152	7	41	H
Dates	2	44	0	0	No
Doughnuts, plain (3″ dia)	1	140	7	45	H
Doughnuts, sugared	1	180	11	55	H
Duck, roast	1 oz	85	6	64	H
Egg:					
Large	1	82	6	64	H
Fried	1	99	8	72	H
Omelet, cheese (2 eggs)	1	334	26	70	H
Eggplant	1 c	38	0	0	No
Eggroll	1	200	11	50	H
Fish cakes	1	162	11	59	H
Flounder, cooked	3 oz	75	1	12	L
Frankfurter, beef	1	176	16	80	H
Frankfurter, chicken	1	116	9	68	H
French toast	1 sl	155	7	41	H
Fruit cocktail, water pack	1/2 c	45	0	0	No
Fruit Pops, frozen	1	70	0	0	No
Grapefruit	1/2	40	0	0	No
Grapefruit juice	4 oz	52	0	0	No
Grapes	10	40	0	0	No
Gravies:					
Au jus, canned	1/3 c	53	1	27	L
Beef, canned	1/4 c	31	2	40	M
Chicken, canned	1/4 c	47	4	65	H

Food	Serving	Calories	Fat Grams	Fat Percentage	Fat Rating
Mushroom, canned	¼ c	30	2	48	M
Greens	½ c	30	0	0	No
Grits, cooked	½ c	62	0	0	No
Haddock, cooked	3 oz	90	1	10	L
Halibut, cooked	3 oz	90	1	10	L
Ham:					
Baked	2 oz	122	6	44	M
Boiled	2 oz	132	6	41	M
Minced	1 oz	75	6	70	H
Herring, pickled	2 oz	126	8	57	M
Honey	1 tbsp	50	0	0	No
Honeydew melon	⅛	62	0	0	No
Ice, fruited	½ c	125	0	0	No
Ice cream (reg)	¼ c	65	4	50	H
Ice cream (rich)	¼ c	82	6	65	H
Ice milk, hard	½ c	100	4	31	M
Ice milk, soft	½ c	133	4	30	M
Jam/jelly	1 tsp	20	0	0	No
Lamb, meat only (no fat)	2 oz	106	4	34	M
Lamb, leg, roasted	1 oz	79	5	62	H
Lard	1 tbsp	115	13	100	H
Lemon	2	40	0	0	No
Lemonade	4 oz	54	0	0	No
Lettuce	2 c	20	0	0	No
Lime	1	40	0	0	No
Liver, calf, cooked	2 oz	148	8	46	M
Lobster meat	3 oz	81	1	14	L
Luncheon meats:					
Barbecue loaf	2 oz	98	6	47	M
Blood sausage	1 oz	107	10	82	H
Bologna, beef	1 oz	89	8	81	H
Bologna, Lebanon	2 oz	128	8	59	M
Braunschweiger	1 oz	102	9	79	H
Chicken roll	2 oz	80	4	44	M
Corned beef loaf	2 oz	92	4	38	M

Food	Serving	Calories	Fat Grams	Fat Percentage	Fat Rating
Ham salad					
spread	1 oz	61	4	65	H
Italian sausage	1 oz	108	9	72	H
Kielbasa	1 oz	88	8	79	H
Knockwurst	1 oz	87	8	81	H
Mortadella	1 oz	88	7	74	H
Pepperoni	1 oz	135	12	80	H
Picnic loaf	1 oz	66	5	64	H
Polish sausage	1 oz	92	8	80	H
Salami	1 oz	128	11	76	H
Smoked link					
sausage	1 oz	112	9	72	H
Thuringer	1 oz	98	9	78	H
Turkey roll	2 oz	84	4	42	M
Vienna sausage	1 oz	80	7	81	H
Macaroni					
noodles, cooked	½ c	75	0	0	No
Macaroni and					
cheese	¼ c	110	6	45	H
Mackerel, cooked	3 oz	101	3	26	L
Mango	½	75	0	0	No
Margarine	1 tsp	36	4	100	H
Mayonnaise	1 tbsp	101	11	100	H
Milk:					
Buttermilk	1 c	88	0.5	2	L
Evaporated,					
unswt.	¼ c	86	5	52	H
Hot chocolate	¼ c	61	3	46	H
Lowfat	½ c	72	2	30	L
Skim	1 c	88	0.5	2	L
Whole	⅓ c	53	3	48	H
Milkshake	⅓ c	120	4	30	M
Muffin	½	100	4	36	H
Mushrooms	1 c	20	0	0	No
Noodles,					
chow mein	½ c	110	6	45	H
Noodles,					
egg, cooked	½ c	100	1	11	L
Oil, vegetable	1 tsp	40	5	100	H

Food	Serving	Calories	Fat Grams	Fat Percentage	Fat Rating
Olives	10	45	5	100	H
Onion	1/2 c	32	0	0	No
Orange	1	45	0	0	No
Orange juice	1/2 c	60	0	0	No
Oysters, whole	10	95	2	24	L
Oysters, meat only	1 c	158	4	24	L
Pancakes (6″ dia)	1	164	5	27	M
Parsnips	1/2 c	70	0	0	No
Paté, all liver	1 oz	90	8	79	H
Peach, fresh	1	38	0	0	No
Peach, halves (in water)	2	56	0	0	No
Peanut butter	1 tbsp	90	8	76	H
Peanuts	1/2 oz	83	7	76	H
Pear, fresh	1/2	50	0	0	No
Pear, halves (in water)	2	60	0	0	No
Peas	1/2 c	50	0	0	No
Pepper, sweet	1 c	24	0	0	No
Pickles:					
Bread and butter	3 sl	16	0	0	No
Dill	1	15	0	0	No
Gherkins (small)	1	22	0	0	No
Sweet relish	1 tbsp	21	0	0	No
Pie, cream	1/8 pie	311	10	28	H
Pie, fruit	1/8 pie	286	13	40	H
Pineapple	1/2 c	40	0	0	No
Pineapple juice	1/2 c	60	0	0	No
Pistachios	1/2 oz	84	8	82	H
Pizza, small, plain	1/8 pie	153	6	32	M
Plums	1	32	0	0	No
Popcorn, no oil	3 c	70	1	13	L
Popcorn, with oil	2 c	80	4	45	H
Popover	1	90	4	35	H
Popsicle	1	90	0	0	No
Pork:					
Loin/chops, no fat	2 oz	144	8	50	M

Food	Serving	Calories	Fat Grams	Fat Percentage	Fat Rating
Roast	1 oz	106	9	76	H
Spareribs	1 oz	126	11	79	H
Potato chips	10	115	8	63	H
Potatoes:					
Au gratin	¼ c	89	5	46	H
Baked	½	70	0	0	No
French fries	5	107	5	42	H
Hash brown	¼ c	89	9	45	H
Mashed with milk/butter	½ c	100	5	45	H
Potato salad	⅓ c	83	4	44	H
Pretzel rods	1	55	0.5	10	L
Prune juice	2 oz	50	0	0	No
Prunes	2	50	0	0	No
Pudding	½ c	192	6	28	M
Quiche Lorraine (9″ dia)	⅛ pie	250	18	65	H
Raisins	2 tbsp	50	0	0	No
Raspberries	½ c	35	0	0	No
Rice, cooked:					
Fried	½ c	180	7	36	H
White/whole grain	½ c	116	0	0	No
Roll, hard (Kaiser)	½	78	1	17	L
Roll, ready to eat	1	119	3	23	M
Salad Dressings:					
Blue cheese	1 tbsp	76	8	95	H
French	1 tbsp	66	6	84	H
Italian	1 tbsp	83	9	98	H
Russian	1 tbsp	74	8	92	H
Salmon	2 oz	104	4	36	M
Sardines, oil packed	1 oz	88	7	72	H
Sauce:					
Barbecue	¼ c	47	1	19	L
Béarnaise (milk/butter)	⅛ c	88	9	88	H
Cheese	¼ c	77	4	50	H
Curry	¼ c	68	4	49	H

Food	Serving	Calories	Fat Grams	Fat Percentage	Fat Rating
Hollandaise	¼ c	59	5	75	H
Stroganoff	¼ c	68	3	35	H
Soy	1 tbsp	11	0	0	No
Sweet & sour	¼ c	75	0	0	No
Tartar	1 tbsp	74	8	100	H
Teriyaki	1 tbsp	15	0	0	No
White	¼ c	60	4	50	H
Scallops	3 oz	95	1	11	L
Seeds, sesame	1 tbsp	47	4	82	H
Seeds, sunflower	¼ c	203	17	75	H
Sherbet	½ c	150	2	12	L
Shrimp, deep fried	2 pc	152	10	57	H
Shrimp, fresh/ frozen	20 med	74	1	10	L
Snow peas	1 c	30	0	0	No
Sole, cooked	3 oz	75	1	12	L
Soups (canned):					
Asparagus, cream of (milk)	1 c	161	8	46	H
Bean with bacon (water)	1 c	173	6	31	M
Bean with ham (ready)	1 c	231	9	33	M
Beef boullion (ready)	1 c	16	.5	30	L
Beef chunky (ready)	1 c	121	5	27	L
Beef noodle (water)	1 c	84	3	33	M
Black bean (water)	1 c	116	1	12	L
Celery, cream of (milk)	1 c	165	10	53	H
Cheese (milk)	1 c	230	15	57	H
Chicken broth (water)	1 c	39	1	32	L
Chicken chunk (ready)	1 c	178	7	34	M

Food	Serving	Calories	Fat Grams	Fat Percentage	Fat Rating
Chicken dumpling (water)	1 c	97	6	51	H
Chicken, cream of (milk)	1 c	191	11	54	H
Chicken gumbo (water)	1 c	56	1	23	M
Chicken noodle (water)	1 c	75	2	29	M
Chicken noodle (ready) with meatballs	1 c	99	4	32	M
Chicken rice (ready)	1 c	127	3	23	L
(water)	1 c	60	2	29	L
Chicken veg. (ready)	1 c	167	5	26	L
(water)	1 c	74	3	35	M
Clam chowder, Manhattan	1 c	133	3	22	L
Clam chowder, New England (milk)	1 c	163	7	36	M
Consommé (water)	1 c	29	0	0	No
Crab (ready)	1 c	76	2	18	L
Escarole (ready)	1 c	27	2	60	H
Gazpacho (ready)	1 c	57	2	35	H
Lentil with ham (ready)	1 c	140	3	18	L
Minestrone (ready)	1 c	127	3	20	L
Mushroom, cream of (milk)	1 c	203	14	60	H
Onion (water)	1 c	57	2	27	M
Oyster stew (milk)	1 c	134	8	53	M
Pea, Green (milk)	1 c	239	7	26	L
Pea, split (ready)	1 c	184	4	19	L

Food	Serving	Calories	Fat Grams	Fat Percentage	Fat Rating
Potato, cream of (milk)	1 c	148	6	39	H
Scotch broth (water)	1 c	80	3	29	M
Shrimp, cream of (milk)	1 c	165	9	57	M
Tomato (water)	1 c	86	2	20	M
Tomato bisque (milk)	1 c	198	7	30	M
Tomato rice (water)	1 c	120	3	20	M
Turkey chunk (ready)	1 c	136	4	29	L
Turkey noodle (water)	1 c	69	2	26	M
Turkey veg. (water)	1 c	74	3	37	H
Vegetable (water)	1 c	72	2	24	M
Vegetable chunk (ready)	1 c	122	4	27	M
Soups (rehydrated)					
Beef bouillon	1 c	19	1	26	M
Beef noodle	1 c	41	1	17	M
Chicken bouillon	1 c	21	1	50	H
Chicken noodle	1 c	53	1	20	M
Leek	1 c	71	2	26	M
Onion	1 c	21	0.5	18	M
Tomato	1 c	102	2	21	M
Vegetable	1 c	55	1	14	L
Spaghetti noodles, ckd	½ c	75	0	0	No
Spinach	1 c	41	0	0	No
Squash, summer	1 c	28	0	0	No
Squash, winter	⅔ c	60	0.5	0	No
Strawberries	1 c	55	0	0	No
Swordfish	3 oz	111	1	14	L
Taco shell	1	140	5.5	35	M
Tangerine	1	39	0	0	No

Food	Serving	Calories	Fat Grams	Fat Percentage	Fat Rating
Tapioca	½ c	110	4	33	M
Tofu	4 oz	80	5	56	M
Tomato	1	27	0	0	No
Tomato juice	1 c	50	0	0	No
Tomatoes, canned	½ c	30	0	0	No
Tomato sauce, jar	¼ c	100	7	63	H
Turnip	1 c	53	0	0	No
Tortilla (6″ dia)	1	70	1	13	L
Tuna, in oil	1 oz	81	6	67	H
Tuna, in water	3 oz	108	1	6	L
Turkey breast	3 oz	93	1	13	L
Veal, cooked	2 oz	133	7	29	M
Waffles	1	86	2	21	M
Walnuts	½ oz	90	9	86	H
Watermelon	1 c	42	0	0	No
Yeast, Brewers	2 tbs	46	0	0	No
Yogurt:					
Plain lowfat	⅔ c	82	3	31	M
Vanilla	½ c	110	2	16	L
Fruited	½ c	120	2	15	L
Plain, whole	½ c	70	4	51	H
Zucchini	1 c	28	0	0	No